THE FOOD ALLERGY DETECTION PROGRAM

THE FOOD ALLERGY DETECTION PROGRAM

Complete With Over 300 Allergen-Free Recipes

TERRY TRAUB

With a Foreword by Stuart M. Bloom, M.D.

FREDERICK FELL PUBLISHERS, INC.
New York, New York

Caution: This book is not intended, nor should it be regarded, as medical advice. When an allergy symptom appears, consult your doctor for the appropriate treatment. In addition, before giving yourself or your child any drug—prescription or over-the-counter—consult your doctor. It is your doctor's function to diagnose the medical problem and prescribe the appropriate medicine, dosage, and course of treatment.

For information address:

Frederick Fell Publishers, Inc.
386 Park Avenue South
New York, New York 10016

Published simultaneously in Canada by Fitzhenry & Whiteside, Limited, Toronto

International Standard Book Number: 0-8119-0592-6
Library of Congress Catalog Card Number: 83-81125

Manufactured in the United States of America

1 2 3 4 5 6 7 8 9 0

To my husband Dave,
and my sons, Garrett and Adam

CONTENTS

FOREWORD

The human species has used the resources of this planet to grow and multiply. Genetics has given us the ability to convert foodstuffs into the building blocks of our bodies—amino acids for proteins, sugars for complex carbohydrates, nucleic acids (DNA and RNA), fats for energy and structure, and minerals for enzymes. These are essential compounds to keep the process going and to allow passage to the next meal.

Our understanding of diet continues to grow, and we often speak of proper dietary habits and food combinations. However, all is not wholesome and palatable in the world. Many compounds are indigestible or downright deadly to everyone. Other potential foodstuffs may be more deleterious to some people than to others through better tolerance or better processing. Furthermore there is the problem of individual, nondeadly sensitivity to our surrounding environment. Most of us are familiar with the concept of an allergy, whether it is caused by grass, food, pollen, or wool. We will, however, restrict this discussion to allergies caused by food alone.

The way an allergy works is that some portion of a foodstuff (usually a protein) provokes the body's defense system to react against unwanted foreigners. This enzyme or toxin that the body reacts to is called an *antigen*. The antibody proteins and the defending white blood cells provide the body's defense against the antigen, thus stimulating an allergic reaction in the person. Our basic antibody system is passed down to us in our genes from our parents, but the system is flexible in its recognition of problem compounds, whether the compounds are viruses, foods, or other dangers.

The reaction of our system is usually speedy and violent when aroused by an allergenic food. Our diet may be liberally studded with foods we are sensitive to, yet we may not realize the nature of our affliction unless careful attention is paid to the details of our encounters. Every point of contact by the antigens does not necessarily yield a reaction; therefore the intensity of symptoms noted by an individual may vary.

We must differentiate this allergic reaction from genetic variations in whole populations that may cause similar symptoms when individuals are challenged by food. (Two prominent examples of the latter are problems related to genetic lack of lactase to digest milk sugar and lack of G-6-P-D enzyme to cope with fava beans.) The book which you are about to use will cover the problem of discovering true allergy to foods that most of us consider our basic right to digest without harm. The care applied to the production of this volume is evident in the great amount of help it will give.

Technology, wealth, and diversity have given us the ability to mix foods without their ingredients being readily apparent. Thus, the consumer often has a hard time understanding what is really eaten. I have seen in my own experience the difficulty in creating awareness of allergic symptoms and in attempting to diagnose the specific cause and create an antigenless diet. Children are beset enough by many of their peers and parents without the additional handicap of being different at the dining table. I know this volume will be of great help to parents faced with difficult dietary choices when cooking for an allergic child. If we can overcome our culturally learned dietary restrictions, the allergic child will eat tastily and happily. One caveat must be added here: children may lose allergic sensitivity as they grow older, therefore, foods may at times be eaten with impunity. When using this book we urge you to consult with your physician or registered dietician because the symptoms of allergy may conceal other illness for which treatment will be very different.

Stuart M. Bloom M.D., A.B.F.P.

PREFACE

The conception of this book came from need. While in the process of determining our son's allergy, my husband and I tried various elimination diets prescribed by our physician. To our dismay our son, Garrett, a good-natured child, started to exhibit negative behavioral changes. For two weeks our household was one of screaming and tantrums. My husband and I, out of desperation, began to research food allergies that may have been causing the manifestations found in our son. The choices were narrowed down to milk or wheat (gluten). We decided on a possible wheat allergy since the symptoms he exhibited did not appear during the period of transition from mother's milk to cow's milk. We then placed our son on a gluten-free diet.

The results were almost immediate. Garrett started gaining weight, his extended abdomen disappeared, his respiratory congestion cleared up, and his diarrhea ceased. All negative behavior disappeared.

Fortunately, my husband and I had been exposed to a broad background of physiology and chemistry in college. This enabled us to bring our knowledge of research procedures and practices to bear on the problem and follow it to a happy conclusion.

Our son Garrett's predicament made me aware that other children and adults may have problems similar to his. They may not have an allergy to wheat, but to some other food. They may be allergic to a combination of foods like my other son, Adam.

With so many elimination diets on the market, why did I feel a new diet was necessary? Simple. Most of these diets did not take into account the problems of the wheat sensitive (gluten) individual. These diets would offer suggestions such as barley cereal (contains gluten) and other similar grains. Also many elimination diets are high in saturated fatty foods, which many allergic individuals cannot absorb. Therefore, the individual undertaking one of these elimination diets may exhibit more negative symptoms than he/she had prior to these diets. Lastly, most of these diets needed revisions to make them more palatable and practical. These problems brought about the concept for this book, one that I consider quite different and unique from other books published on the subject.

The purpose of this book is not to diagnose whether the reaction to a particular food is caused by malabsorption, intolerance, or a true food allergy, nor is it the book's purpose to suggest treatment. This belongs to the realm of the physician. Rather, the intent is to help the allergic (for lack of a better word) individual or parent of the individual to discover the cause of their physical distress after the ingestion of food, and to reduce the culinary hardships for those who must deal with the problem. Once the offending food or foods are discovered and noted, this information will aid the physician in proper diagnosis and treatment.

There are a great number of other food-associated allergies that this book does not address. Allergies caused by food additives, chemical sprays, and drug interaction can also enter into the picture.

Terry Traub

ACKNOWLEDGMENTS

This book was influenced by the suggestions and encouragement of many people.

I would like to express my gratitude to Dr. Stuart Bloom, who examined my manuscript for its medical accuracy, for all his aid and support toward the completion of this book.

Thank you to my mother, Mary Thurston, for all her work and effort. I would like to say a special thank you to Mrs. Denise McBreen for her special help and expertise in forming the recipe section of this book.

My thanks to the many recipe contributors. These include: Doris Thurston, Shirley Porter, Georgette Davis, David Traub, Lauri Geoghegan, Dick McCaughy, Sue Ann White, Lilian Garvin, Stephanie Cole, Diane Goldstein, and Muriel Eastwood.

PART I

INTRODUCTION

The ingestion of food is normally a simple, satisfying process to most people. However, many individuals, especially children, may exhibit abnormal or exaggerated reactions to food. These reactions manifest themselves in a variety of ways and can cause much discomfort. They are generally called food hypersensitivity or simple food allergy. Symptoms of food allergies in children can take the form of runny noses, coughing, itchy throat, wheezing, diarrhea, abdominal pain, excessive sweating, mucus in the chest, eczema, constipation, and vomiting. In adults, the symptoms of food allergies may take the form of hayfever, asthma, diarrhea, eczema, headache, dizziness, eye problems, and others frequently confused with other diseases. Such a variety in symptoms and the time period involved for reaction to the food by the individual makes immediate diagnosis by the physician almost impossible.

Food allergies may be temporary, permanent, or delayed. Temporary food allergies will disappear after a period of abstinence and slow reintroduction. A permanent allergy is a fixed allergy which will not disappear even after years of avoidance. Masked allergy or delayed allergy is a latent reaction to a food. This reaction can take anywhere from twelve to seventy-two hours to manifest itself after the ingestion of a food (wheat especially is known to have this property of delayed reaction).

Some allergies to food seem to be more prominent at certain times of the year. This seems to be due to two reasons. First, many foods are seasonal and are available in higher quantities at certain times. Secondly, some allergies have properties that when combined with a certain food during a pollinating time of the year may produce a reaction, while ingestion of the food during the nonpollinating season produces no reaction. The following chart indicates common allergy manifestations.

ALLERGY MANIFESTATIONS

Symptoms	Diarrhea and Gastric Distress	Migraines	Headaches	Eczema
Possible Food Causes	Wheat and gluten-related foods (oats, barley, rye) Raw meat Pineapple juice Citrus juices Milk Beer, gin, whiskey	Monosodium Glutamate Salt (even a small amount) Cheese (yellow especially) Chocolate Cokes, colas Ham Milk products Nuts (especially coconuts) Pineapple Alcohol: beer, wine (especially red), bourbon, scotch, liqueurs and brandy (very potent)	Same as migraines Caffeine (in tea and coffee) Refined sugar Wheat	Milk

Symptoms	Hives (Articaria) and Itching	Swelling	Anaphylactic Shock	Sinus and Nasal Congestion	Asthma
Possible Food Causes	Chocolate Fruits such as strawberries, oranges, tomatoes	Honey Eggs (egg whites)	Egg whites	Milk Cheese Meats Chocolate Sauerkraut Wines and beer	Many foods —list may be endless Usually complicated by stress factors and other allergies to pollens and grasses

CAUSES OF FOOD ALLERGIES

The etiology and mechanics of food allergies is not fully understood. Frequent confusion takes place between food allergy and food intolerance making proper diagnosis of the problem difficult.

Food allergy is an immediate abnormal reaction to ingestion of the food. Such reactions take the form of asthma, hives, migraine, and acute anaphylactic attacks.

Food intolerance is an exaggerated but not immediate reaction by the body that suggests a relationship to food. Symptoms of intolerance that develop after eating a specific food are eczema, diarrhea, migraines, stomach distress, and vomiting. Many foods such as apples, melons, cucumbers, onions, garlic, boiled cabbage, coconuts, coffee, and many spices are known for their difficulty in digestion. If the individual is lacking the proper enzyme to hydrolyze the food, then the food is not properly digested, but rather excreted by the body in the form of diarrhea with stomach pain. Ingestion by children and adults of certain sugars (i.e., lactose in milk) and certain carbohydrates may cause diarrhea.

Food allergies are due to sensitivity developed after exposure to a food. Sometimes it is the simple proteins in the food that are the trouble-makers. In milk, it is casein, laceatbumin, and/or lactoglobulin; in eggs, it is usually ovalbumin found in the egg white; in wheat, it is either gluten or gliadin; and in corn, it is zein.

Another type of food-related difficulty that causes frequent confusion is the malabsorption syndrome found with celiac disease in children and tropical sprue in adults. Its symptoms resemble food intolerance symptoms due to the diarrhea and gastric distress exhibited by the individual. This disease is caused by the ingestion of the cereal protein, gluten. This protein, found mainly in wheat, is also found in oats, rye, and barley. The mechanics of this disease have not been established, although it is known that the fraction of gluten, gliadin, initiates the changes in the lining of the intestine. It is also hypothesized that the disease is gene-related. Negative results of this wasting disease include loss of weight, runting, swelling of the abdomen, and dehydration.

Food allergies may occur at any age and at any time from infancy to adulthood. Scientists have found that unchanged proteins absorbed into the bloodstream can be passed by the placenta. These scientists theorize that sensitivity may develop while the fetus is in the mother's womb, or by the transmission of the sensitivity in the mother's milk.

TESTING FOR FOOD ALLERGIES

There are various methods of testing for food allergies. Some examples are:

1. The Skin Test. This is a method by which a suspected antigen is introduced to the body by scratching the skin, by intradermal injection, or by applying it to the surface of the skin and covering it. While skin testing is quite reliable for discovering allergies to grasses, dusts, and pollens, it is an unreliable test for food allergy. This is due to the difficulties encountered in the preparation of the numerous food extracts and the instability of the extracts once they are prepared.
2. Serum or Blood Test. Radioallergosorbent test (RAST) is an unreliable diagnostic tool for everyone, except those individuals that have immediate allergic reactions. Like the skin test, it is known to give false positives to foods tested.
3. Fasting. This type of test is performed *only* under the supervision of a physician and usually the individual is hospitalized. The patient goes on a water diet for 4 to 6 days while receiving numerous blood tests. Then single foods are added at prescribed intervals and any reaction is noted. This procedure continues for a two-week period. This is one of the better methods of food allergy detection, but the expense of this type of investigation and the occasional physiological side-effects restrict its use.
4. Chemically Defined Elemental Diets. This test involves the administration of fluids containing essential nutrients while eliminating all solids. This is performed in the hospital under the supervision of a physician.
5. Elimination Diet. This is a nonallergic diet the individual may ingest without the necessity of fasting or the usage of the elemental diet. An individual eats 5 items a day, such as pineapple for breakfast, millet cereal for lunch with milk, and turkey and carrots for dinner. Each day more items are added and a diary is kept of any reactions. This type of elimination diet has been utilized by physicians for more than 35 years. However, due to new methods of food preparation and the heavy reliance on additives, sweeteners, and preservatives of food packagers in today's market, the food items listed in this type of elimination diet are no longer truly hypoallergenic. These diets are also extremely bland and it is difficult to stick to such a diet. Most failures today in elimination diets are due to the individual's inability to adhere to the diet.

THE ELIMINATION DIET: HOW IT WORKS

There is general disagreement on which foods cause the most allergies. However, most allergists agree that milk, eggs, corn, wheat (gluten), chocolate, citrus fruits, and pork are primarily responsible for food-related allergies. These foods, along with all prepared foods, will be eliminated in the diet that follows. These foods will then be reintroduced individually over a period of time in order to discover and record any abnormal reactions.

All of the above foods mentioned will be eliminated for twelve days. These twelve days are subdivided into four day sections with a *turkey day*, a *fish day*, a *vegetarian day*, and a *lamb day*, named for the main focus food of each day. These foods and others will be ingested in sequence. Strict adherence to the sequence is important for elimination and identification of *all* offending foods.

After the twelve days, the individual will then add the first suspected food (for example, milk) to his elimination diet for three days. This time frame will ensure maximum results. He will simultaneously keep a diary of any possible symptoms. The individual will then return for four days to the original elimination diet until it can be assumed that this food (milk) is not the cause of the food allergy.

If, however, any reactions are noted up to three days following the ingestion of milk, these reactions will be noted along with the time of the reaction. This procedure will be followed until all suspected foods are tested. You should consult your doctor for treatment of any unusual or persistent allergy symptoms. Tests must be made in this order: milk, eggs, gluten, corn, chocolate, citrus fruits, and pork.

The individual should note that in this new elimination diet, no food family is eaten consistently three days in a row except for rice, lettuce, and other foods known to be hypoallergenic. This is an important feature of the elimination diet for the individual to note and continue to be aware of. By separating the food families each day, an allergy to a particular food family can be easily identified. If the individual is not able to find or acquire the correct food item described in the elimination diet, he may choose an alternative, listed in the column next to the menu column. An example would be: Day 1 suggests apricots for breakfast. Apricots belong to the plum family, therefore, the individual may select any fruit from that family. Those belonging to the plum family are: plums, cherries, peaches, or nectarines. All fruits must be peeled if fresh, or packed in their own juices if canned. Fruit canned in syrup is NOT allowed until the individual is tested for corn allergies. All dishes marked with asterisks (*) have recipes in the book and can be located by consulting the index.

PREPARATION FOR THE ELIMINATION DIET

Due to the fact that *no* prepared foods may be included in this diet, alternative stock items for the pantry will be needed.

[7]

Beans
    Pinto (kidney)
    Garbanzo beans (chickpeas)
    Lentils

Beef
    Kosher meats (always without milk products)
    Lean beef

Cereals
    Puffed rice
    Puffed millet

Cheese
    Cheeses made from goat's milk
    Cheeses made from ewe's milk (sheep)
    (See Ingredient Glossary)

Eggs
    Jolly Joan Egg Replacer (not milk-free)
    Golden Harvest Egg Replacer (not milk-free)
    Unflavored gelatin
    Baking powder (cereal-free/egg-free)

Fish
    Canned salmon (fifteen-ounce can)
    Canned tuna (seven-ounce can packed in its own oil or fresh water)

Flour
    Tapioca flour
    Potato flour
    Potato starch
    Rice flour
    Rice baking mix (gluten-free)
    Arrowroot flour
    Soy flour

Fruit
    Fresh or canned in its own juices. (Do not buy canned fruit in either heavy or light syrup.)

Grains
    Brown rice
    Enriched white rice
    Risotto
    Millet
    Buckwheat groats (Kasha)

Liquids
    Soy milk (Soyamel and others)
    Bottled water
    Non-citrus juices
    Herb teas (without caffeine)

Mayonnaise
    Eggless mayonnaise (Hains brand or Featherweight)

Meats
    Lamb

Nuts
    Almonds
    Pine nuts

Oils and Margarines
    Safflower oil and/or margarine
    Sesame seed oil
    Soybean oil or margarine
    Olive oil (use sparingly)

Poultry
    Tom turkey (if chicken, always males)

Seasonings and Spices
    Rice miso (rice oriental seasoning)
    Sea salt
    Herbs and spices
    Tamari

Soybean
    Tofu

Sweeteners
    Carob
    Honey
    Blackstrap molasses

Preliminary Cooking

If the individual begins the elimination diet on a Sunday, for example, certain sauces, dressings, and beverages need to be prepared prior to initiating the diet. This advanced preparation will allow the cook more time and less work during the execution of the diet. Some items that should be prepared before diet initiation are:

1. Two loafs of rice bread (yeast-raised)
2. Roquefort Dressing* (needs two days of refrigeration prior to serving)
3. French Dressing*
4. Riceola*
5. Homemade Maple Syrup*
6. Homemade Mayonnaise*

Foods NOT allowed on this elimination diet:

Wheat
Oats
Barley
Rye
Corn
Corn syrup (found in most canned fruit—check label)
Citrus fruits
Pineapple
Pork
     bacon
     ham
Eggs
Chocolate
Coffee (not in any form)
Tea (unless decaffeinated); herb teas are okay
Wine
Alcohol
Beer
Ale
Cinnamon
Cow's milk (sheep's and goat's milk allowed)
Cheese (sheep's and goat's milk cheese allowed)
Nuts—all except almonds
Chewing gum
Margarines containing corn or milk products
Crustaceans of any form—lobster, crab, shrimp
Monosodium glutamate (known to cause migraines)

QUESTIONS AND ANSWERS

1. *Do I need to strictly stay on the diet?* Yes, straying off the diet will produce different results, thereby invalidating the information gathered during the diet.

2. *Can I eat at restaurants?* No, most restaurants use milk, eggs, and wheat-based flour in their cooking.

3. *What if I'm allergic to turkey or fish?* This diet provides two substitutes for those who may be allergic to either turkey or fish. Beef may be substituted for turkey and chicken may be substituted for fish. Check Appendix B.

4. *Will I spend much time in the kitchen?* If you prepare the essentials prior to starting the diet as explained in the previous pages, the time spent in the kitchen should be about normal.

5. *Where do I find the ingredients necessary for the diet?* Generally, most health food stores carry all the ingredients listed as necessary in this diet. If not, ask the store to special order the item for you.

6. *Should I take vitamin supplements during this diet?* Ask your doctor for advice on vitamins. If he does consider them necessary, be careful of the vitamins you buy. Some manufacturers use cornstarch as a binder, others use fish oil in the mixture. Read the label!

7. *What if I'm allergic to something in the elimination diet?* This is not an unusual occurrence. Many people have been known to be allergic to the control serum in skin tests. If you find you are allergic to something in the elimination diet, it will not be difficult to discover which food it is. The food families are ingested in sequence. Just check your food chart for which days the symptoms appear and narrow it down. Once you have found the allergen, note it, take it out of the elimination diet, and replace it with another food family that you know you are not allergic to.

8. *Do I have to prepare the meats any special way?* Yes, all chicken and turkey recipes should not include any skin.

9. *Can I substitute shortening or butter for margarine in any of the recipes?* First let's get our terms straight. Shortening is a universal term for solidified vegetable oils, lard, salt pork, beef or lamb. The flavor variety obtained from the various forms of shortening is due to fatty acids. Saturated fatty acids that are usually a solid at room temperature come from animal sources. Unsaturated fatty acids, including polyunsaturates, are generally liquid at room temperature. These are cold-pressed vegetable oils. Hydrogenated vegetable shortening is an unsaturated vegetable oil that has had hydrogen added to it to change it from liquid to solid. Doing so changes the oil from unsaturated to saturated. Even so-called polyunsaturated cubed margarines only contain 30–40 percent polyunsaturated fatty acids.

So now to answer the question. No, you may not use shortening in place of margarine if it is saturated, whether animal or vegetable. Why? because wheat-sensitive people cannot absorb solid fats but liquid oils are readily absorbed. And while a person is on the elimination diet, all sources of irritation need to be covered.

THE ELIMINATION DIET

DAY 1—TURKEY DAY

Menu	Food Family and Substitute	Time Ingested	Symptoms	Time of Symptoms
Breakfast				
Rice Pancakes*	Grass family—no substitutes allowed			
Maple Syrup*	Maple family			
Fresh apricots	Plum family—nectarines, peaches, cherries (not canned in corn syrup)			
Lunch				
Nutty Fruit Salad*	Plum family			
Dessert (optional)				
Beverage				
Dinner				
Turkey Gravy*	Grass family			
Turkey roasted and stuffed*	Fowl family—chicken, but not recommended			
Rice Stuffing*	Grass family			
Cranberry sauce	Blueberry family			
Dessert (optional)				
Beverage				

NOTE: Cut remaining turkey into: (1) slices for sandwiches; (2) slices for hot turkey sandwiches; (3) cubes for turkey salad or soup. Freeze these portions until the next turkey day.

NOTE: All dishes marked with asterisks (*) have recipes in the book and can be located by consulting the index.

DAY 2—FISH DAY

Menu	Food Family and Substitute	Time Ingested	Symptoms	Time of Symptoms
Breakfast				
Riceola*	Grass family—millet			
Banana	Banana family			
Cranberry juice	Blueberry family			
Lunch				
Tuna sandwich* (may use Eggless Mayonnaise I* and lettuce)	Fish family			

Menu	Food Family and Substitute	Time Ingested	Symptoms	Time of Symptoms
Pears	Apple family—fresh apples, crabapple, quince			
Dessert (optional)				
Beverage				
Dinner				
Oven-Baked Fish*	Fish family—snapper, cod			
Green Salad*	Composite family—endive, etc.			
Roquefort Dressing*	Meat family—made from lamb's milk			
French Fries*	Nightshade family			
Beverage				

DAY 3—VEGETARIAN DAY

Menu	Food Family and Substitute	Time Ingested	Symptoms	Time of Symptoms
Breakfast				
Apricot Nut Bread*	Plum family			
Cantaloupe	Gourd family			
Beverage				
Lunch				
Lentil Soup*	Pea family—lentils			
Rice Bread*	Grass family			
Fresh carrots	Parsley family			
Beverage				
Dinner				
Vegeburger*	Pea family			
Artichoke-Spinach Salad*	Goosefoot and composite families			
Dessert (optional)				
Beverage				

DAY 4—LAMB DAY

Menu	Food Family and Substitute	Time Ingested	Symptoms	Time of Symptoms
Breakfast				
Cooked millet	Grass family—rice (puffed or cooked)			
Maple Syrup*	Maple family			
Blueberries	Blueberry family—cranberries			

DAY 4—LAMB DAY (continued)

Menu	Food Family and Substitute	Time Ingested	Symptoms	Time of Symptoms
Beverage				
Lunch				
Beet Salad*	Goosefoot family—chard and composite family			
French Dressing*				
Dessert (optional)				
Beverage				
Dinner				
Lamb Kabob*	Meat family			
Dessert				
Beverage				

DAY 5—TURKEY DAY

Menu	Food Family and Substitute	Time Ingested	Symptoms	Time of Symptoms
Breakfast				
Waffles*	Grass family			
Maple Syrup*	Maple family			
Peaches	Plum family			
Beverage				
Lunch				
Turkey sandwiches	Fowl family and grass family			
Cranberries	Blueberry family			
Dessert (optional)				
Beverage				
Dinner				
Hot Turkey Sandwiches*	Fowl family			
Rice Bread*	Grass family			
Brussel sprouts	Mustard family			
Dessert (optional)				
Beverage				

DAY 6—FISH DAY

Menu	Food Family and Substitute	Time Ingested	Symptoms	Time of Symptoms
Breakfast				
Rice Pancakes*	Grass family			
Maple Syrup*	Maple family			
Beverage				
Lunch				
French Onion Soup*	Lily family			
Potato Salad*	Nightshade family			
Fresh apples	Apple family			
Beverage				
Dinner				
New Orleans Snapper*	Fish family			
Rice	Grass family			
Green Salad*	Composite family			
Dessert (optional)				
Beverage				

DAY 7—VEGETARIAN DAY

Menu	Food Family and Substitute	Time Ingested	Symptoms	Time of Symptoms
Breakfast				
Cooked buckwheat	Buckwheat family			
Maple Syrup*	Maple family			
Apricots	Plum family			
Beverage				
Lunch				
Avocado Provençal Salad*	Laurel family			
Sliced cucumber	Gourd family			
Dessert (optional)				
Beverage				
Dinner				
Pinto Chili*	Pea family			
Zucchini	Gourd family			
Dessert (optional)				
Beverage				

[*15*]

DAY 8—LAMB DAY

Menu	Food Family and Substitute	Time Ingested	Symptoms	Time of Symptoms
Breakfast				
Cooked millet	Grass family			
Maple Syrup*	Maple family			
Cranberries	Blueberry family			
Beverage				
Lunch				
Artichoke-Spinach Salad*	Goosefoot and composite families			
Fresh cauliflower	Mustard family			
Beverage				
Dinner				
Easy Lamb Casserole*	Meat family			
Cooked beets	Goosefoot family			
Dessert (optional)				
Beverage				

DAY 9—TURKEY DAY

Menu	Food Family and Substitute	Time Ingested	Symptoms	Time of Symptoms
Breakfast				
Riceola*	Grass family			
Peaches	Plum family			
Beverage				
Lunch				
Turkey Rice Soup*	Fowl family			
Green salad	Composite family			
French Dressing*				
Dessert (optional)				
Beverage				
Dinner				
Radishes and cauliflower	Mustard family			
Turkey Salad*	Fowl family			
Dessert (optional)				
Beverage				

DAY 10—FISH DAY

Menu	Food Family and Substitute	Time Ingested	Symptoms	Time of Symptoms
Breakfast				
Apple Nut Coffee Cake*	Apple and plum families			
Lunch				
Tuna Patties*	Fish family			
Banana	Banana family			
Dessert (optional)				
Beverage				
Dinner				
Salmon Pie*	Fish and grass families			
Green Salad*	Composite family			
French Dressing*				
Dessert (optional)				
Beverage				

DAY 11—VEGETARIAN DAY

Menu	Food Family and Substitute	Time Ingested	Symptoms	Time of Symptoms
Breakfast				
Cooked millet	Grass family			
Maple Syrup*	Maple family			
Honeydew melon	Gourd family			
Beverage				
Lunch				
Cream of Celery Soup*	Parsley family			
Potato Salad*	Nightshade family			
Apples	Apple family			
Beverage				
Dinner				
Zucchini Boats*	Gourd family			
Rice Bread*	Grass family			
Carrot-Raisin Salad*	Parsley and grape family			
Dessert (optional)				
Beverage				

[*17*]

Menu	Food Family and Substitute	Time Ingested	Symptoms	Time of Symptoms
Breakfast				
Rice Pancakes*	Grass family			
Maple Syrup*	Maple family			
Blueberries	Blueberry family			
Beverage				
Lunch				
Beet Salad*	Goosefoot family			
Banana	Banana family			
Dessert (optional)				
Beverage				
Dinner				
Lamb Stuffed in Grape Leaves*	Meat and grass families			
Green Salad*	Composite family			
French Dressing*				
Dessert (optional)				
Beverage				

TESTING FOR MILK, EGGS, WHEAT, AND CORN

To test for a food allergy, one must challenge the suspected offending food. The elimination diet must still be followed, adding only the suspected food for three days, then returning to the elimination diet for four days. Refer to Recommended Recipes for Testing for menu ideas during testing.

Testing for Milk

For three days, add cow's milk products.
Examples: Cottage cheese for breakfast; cheese for lunch; Turkey Goulash* for dinner; Vegetarian Pizza* for the vegetarian dinner.
Return to the elimination diet for four days.

Testing for Eggs

For three days, add eggs.
Examples: Eggs (fried, scrambled, etc.) for breakfast; add egg to bread recipes; egg salads for lunch; egg omelets and eggs as binders in recipes for dinner; use eggs in Salmon Pie.*
Return to the elimination diet for four days.

Testing for Wheat

For three days, add wheat products.

Examples: When making homemade bread (see recipes), use wheat flour as a base instead of the flours stated; have wheat toast and waffles made from wheat flour for breakfast; have homemade bread for lunch; choose Chicken Divan* for dinner and meatless spaghetti for vegetarian day.

Return to the elimination diet for four days. This is especially important for wheat allergy testing. Wheat allergies are known to be masked allergies with latent symptoms of up to 72 hours.

Testing for Corn

For three days, add corn products.

Examples: Add corn syrup to the maple syrup for breakfast; add creamed corn or fresh corn at lunch and dinner; choose Deep Fried Fish* for dinner.

Return to the elimination diet for four days.

Follow the same procedure for chocolate, citrus fruits, pork, and any other suspected allergen.

TESTING FOR MILK WORKSHEET

Menu	Food Family and Substitute	Time Ingested	Symptoms	Time of Symptoms
Breakfast				
Lunch				
Dinner				

TESTING FOR EGGS WORKSHEET

Menu	Food Family and Substitute	Time Ingested	Symptoms	Time of Symptoms
Breakfast				
Lunch				
Dinner				

TESTING FOR WHEAT WORKSHEET

Menu	Food Family and Substitute	Time Ingested	Symptoms	Time of Symptoms
Breakfast				
Lunch				
Dinner				

[20]

Menu	Food Family and Substitute	Time Ingested	Symptoms	Time of Symptoms
Breakfast				
Lunch				
Dinner				

SOURCES OF MILK, EGGS, WHEAT, AND CORN

A great deal of research and label reading is necessary to eliminate all allergy sources. The following lists include examples of foods containing allergens. These are not complete lists for foods, for manufacturing techniques are forever changing.

Sources of Milk (Cow's)

milk—whole, low-fat, skimmed
milk—condensed
milk—powdered and evaporated
buttermilk
creams—sour and whipped
ice cream
ice milk
milk chocolate
cheeses (except those made from ewe's, goat's, reindeer's or buffalo's milk)
creamed foods
scrambled eggs
butter
some margarines

pie crusts
cookies
Bisquick and pancake mixes
crackers
biscuits
doughnuts
bavarians and mousses
souffles
au gratin foods
soups
bologna
sausage
nougat
fritters

Sources of Eggs

malted chocolate drinks
frostings and icings
Hollandaise sauce
custards
french toast
glazed rolls
hamburger mix
mayonnaise
marshmallows
meringues
creamed pies
eggnog
ice cream
noodles

macaroni
jelly rolls
doughnuts
Bisquick
pancake and waffle mixes
salad dressings
souffles
bavarians and mousses
tartar sauce
sausages
sherbets
breads
cakes

Sources of Wheat

beer, ale
gin, whiskey
malted beverages
rolls
doughnuts
crackers
cookies
biscuits
pretzels
commercial cornbread
commercial millet breads
gluten flour and breads
farina
rye
oats
graham
wheat starch

flours—all-purpose, white
flours—wheat, enriched
bran products
pumpernickel
wheat germ
wheat cereals
chocolate candy bars
commercial gravy mixes†
puddings
sausages
bologna
matzo
Bisquick and pancake mixes
some yeasts
some ice creams
noodles, spaghetti
vermicelli

†Some commercial gravy mixes use potato starch as their base.
NOTE: Most wheat-free flours such as soy, millet, corn, and potato, are usually mixed with wheat flours in commercial breads.

Sources of Corn

beer, ale
gin, whiskey
carbonated drinks
instant tea
instant coffee
soybean milk and formula†
ice cream
sherbets
custards
puddings
Jell-O
commercial cakes and cookies
doughnuts
confectioners sugar
commercial pie crusts
non-dairy creamers†
non-dairy whipped toppings†
frostings
popcorn
caramel coloring

catsup
baking powder†
crackers
fruit canned in syrup
confection dates
corn cereals
jams
jellies
canned soups
tortillas
salad dressings†
syrups
monosodium glutamate
corn chips
hominy
chili
hot dogs
peanut butter
nuts
cornstarch

†Some brands do not contain corn.
NOTE: Cornstarch is used as a base in many brands of aspirin, vitamins, toothpastes, and glue. A corn base is found in most paper products such as wax paper and paper cartons.

PART II
ALLERGY COOKBOOK

INTRODUCTION

When first faced with the fact that convenience foods, basic grains, and dairy products cannot be used in menu planning, any cook would be dismayed. But with a little practice, patience, and planning, all problems can be overcome.

The object of this recipe section is to guide the cook into a new era of discovery. Not all allergy cookery is bland and unattractive; in fact, just the opposite. Many foods throughout the world are inherently hypo-allergenic.

This recipe section includes recipes that were invented by and gathered from our grandparents and ancestors, and adjusted for the modern kitchen. Also included are recipes researched from lands that are known to have few food allergies, like Japan. It is hoped that the cook using this book will consider these recipes and cooking methods an adventure.

LEGEND

The recipes in this cookbook are coded in three different ways:

1. Those recipes that are safe to eat during the elimination diet and afterwards for maintenance will be marked with the letter E. The recipe will have the following under the title: E (milkless, eggless, glutenless, cornless).
2. Those recipes to be used during the testing period will be marked with the letter T, for example: T (testing for eggs—milkless, gluten-less, cornless).
3. Those recipes that simply state what they do not contain. They will list the eliminated ingredients under the title, such as milkless, glutenless, or cornless.

(All dishes marked with asterisks (*) are located in the book and can be found by consulting the index.)

APPETIZERS AND DIPS

AVOCADO COCKTAIL DELIGHT

E (*milkless, eggless, glutenless, cornless*)

3 tomatoes, peeled and diced
2 small, ripe avocados
½ teaspoon sweet basil
2 tablespoons chopped fresh
   parsley
2 tablespoons pine nuts
2 tablespoons minced shallots
2 tablespoons lemon juice (omit
   during elimination diet)
2 tablespoons olive oil
   Salt and pepper to taste

Peel, dice tomatoes, and discard seeds. Dice avocados. Gently combine basil, parsley, and pine nuts with tomatoes and avocado. In a separate small mixing bowl, mix together shallots, lemon juice, olive oil, salt, and pepper, and pour over combined vegetables. Serve immediately in chilled cocktail glasses.

Serves 6

CAPONATA

E (*milkless, eggless, glutenless, cornless*)

2 medium eggplants, unpeeled,
cut into 1-inch cubes
¾ cup olive oil
2 large onions, chopped
2 small zucchini, unpeeled, sliced
½ cup chopped green pepper
1 cup chopped celery
1 cup chopped fresh tomatoes

2 tablespoons capers
⅓ cup red wine vinegar
2 tablespoons brown sugar
¼ cup chopped fresh basil, or
1 teaspoon dried basil
2 tablespoons pine nuts
¼ cup chopped parsley
Pepper

In a large skillet, brown eggplant in olive oil. Remove and set aside. Add onions, celery, zucchini, and green pepper and sauté until tender. Add tomatoes and cook until tender. Add eggplant, capers, vinegar, sugar, basil, and nuts. Cover and simmer for 10 minutes. Chill and serve on toasted bread. Garnish with parsley and pepper.

Serves 8

GUACAMOLE DIP

E (*milkless, eggless, glutenless, cornless*)

3 to 4 ripe avocados, skinned and
seeds removed
½ cup finely chopped onion
⅛ teaspoon minced garlic
½ teaspoon salt

½ cup stewed tomatoes
1 teaspoon vinegar
3 tablespoons tomato paste
1 small can green chiles, chopped
(use less for a mild dip)

Mash avocados into a paste. Add all other ingredients. Mix well. Chill before serving.

HUMMUS DIP

E (*milkless, eggless, glutenless, cornless*)

1 cup canned garbanzo beans
⅔ cup Tahini Sauce*
1 tablespoon chopped parsley

Press garbanzo beans through a sieve or purée in a blender or food processor until smooth, but not too thick. Slowly add purée to Tahini Sauce. Chill. Serve topped with chopped parsley.

Serves 6

NOTE: This is good with fresh vegetables.

ORIENTAL SALMON TOFU DIP

E (*milkless, eggless, glutenless, cornless*)

1 can salmon (7¾ oz.), drained and flaked
¼ cup sliced shallots
½ cup tofu, mashed
½ cup Eggless Mayonnaise I*

2 teaspoons tamari (traditional/ wheat-free)
¼ teaspoon ground ginger
1 tablespoon toasted sesame seeds
Vegetables of choice, sliced

In a medium-size mixing bowl combine all ingredients except vegetables. Mix well with a whisk. Chill for 2 hours. Serve with vegetables.

FRIED TOFU

E (*milkless, eggless, glutenless, cornless*)

1 cup tamari (traditional wheat-free) with miso
3 tablespoons milkless margarine
1 jar pimento (2½ oz.), finely chopped
1 pound fresh tofu, sliced

Soak tofu in tarmari for 2 hours. Melt margarine in a skillet, add tofu slices and fry quickly on both sides. Sprinkle with chopped pimento.

Serves 8

GREEK FRIED CHEESE I

E (*milkless, eggless, glutenless, cornless*)

3 tablespoons milkless margarine
¼ cup chopped fresh parsley

1 pound Feta or Kassari cheese,
sliced

Melt margarine in a large skillet. Over medium high heat, fry cheese slices quickly on each side until golden brown. Sprinkle with parsley. Serve hot.

Serves 8

GREEK FRIED CHEESE II

E (*milkless, eggless, glutenless, cornless*)

½ pound Kassari or Kefalotysi
cheese (imported/sheep)
Flour (soy or potato)

Juice of 1 lemon
1 tablespoon oregano

Cut slices of cheese ½ inch thick. Dust with flour and fry in very hot margarine for 30 seconds on each side. Sprinkle with lemon juice and oregano. Serve hot on beds of lettuce and sliced tomato.

Serves 4

KASSARI CHEESE ROLLS

E (*milkless, eggless, glutenless, cornless*)

1 cup soy flour
1 cup potato starch
1 teaspoon salt
2 tablespoons baking powder
3 tablespoons sugar

½ cup milkless margarine
1 cup water
1½ cup grated Kassari cheese
(imported/sheep)

Sift day ingredients twice. Add margarine and water and mix well. Stir in grated cheese. Form batter into rolls and chill for 1 to 2 hours. Place rolls on a greased cookie sheet and bake at 375–400° for 20–25 minutes. Serve hot.

Makes 10–12 rolls

TASTY MEATBALLS

E (*milkless, eggless, glutenless, cornless*)

Meatballs:
1 pound lean ground beef
1 egg substitute (see Appendix A)
½ cup finely diced onion
¾ cup crushed brown rice snaps
¼ cup soy baby formula
    (concentrate and cornless)
1 tablespoon tamari (traditional/
    wheat-free)
¼ teaspoon garlic salt
½ teaspoon tumeric
¼ teaspoon salt
⅛ teaspoon pepper

Sauce:
½ cup Beef Stock*
¼ cup soy baby formula
2 tablespoons tamari
3 tablespoons safflower oil

Mix meatball ingredients together until thoroughly combined. Form mixture into 1-inch meatballs. Sauté meatballs in oil until just brown. Add beef stock. Cover and simmer 12 minutes or until meatballs are cooked through.

Set aside meatballs on a warm platter. Add soy formula and tamari to broth. Stir until thickened. Place meatballs on a platter and pour sauce over them.

Serves 15

GIANT STUFFED MUSHROOMS I

E (*milkless, eggless, glutenless, cornless*)

10–15 huge fresh mushrooms
¼ cup milkless margarine, melted
2 tablespoons chopped shallots,
    or scallions
2 tablespoons milkless margarine
2 teaspoons sweet rice flour,
    arrowroot, or tapioca flour

½ cup non-dairy creamer (cornless
    variety, see Appendix A under *Milk*)
3 tablespoons chopped fresh
    parsley
2 tablespoons Romano cheese,
    grated (imported/sheep)
Salt and pepper to taste

Wash mushrooms. Remove stems and reserve. Dry caps, brush them with melted margarine and arrange, hollow side up, in a baking dish. Chop stems, and by handfuls twist in a corner of a towel to extract as much juice as possible. Sauté with the shallots or scallions in margarine for 4 to 5 minutes. Lower heat and add flour. Add non-dairy creamer and simmer until thickened. Stir in parsley, salt, and pepper. Fill the mushroom caps with this mixture and top each with one teaspoon of Romano.

Bake for 15 minutes or so in upper third of a 375° oven until caps are tender and stuffing is lightly browned.

Serves 10–15

STUFFED MUSHROOMS II

E (*milkless, eggless, glutenless, cornless*)

12 large fresh mushrooms
½ cup chopped onion
1 garlic clove, minced
3 tablespoons milkless margarine
3 tablespoons rice bran
3 tablespoons rice bread,*
   crumbled

¼ cup chopped sunflower seeds
1 tablespoon chopped fresh
   parsley
Salt and pepper to taste
¼ teaspoon hot pepper sauce
2 tablespoons grated Romano
   cheese (imported/sheep)

Clean mushrooms. Remove stems and chop. Set caps aside. Sauté onion, garlic, and chopped stems in a large skillet with melted margarine. Add bran crumbs, sunflower seeds, parsley, salt, pepper, and pepper sauce. Stuff caps with mixture and sprinkle Romano cheese on top. Place mushrooms on a cookie sheet and bake at 400° for 10 minutes. Serve hot.

Serves 12

ROQUEFORT STUFFED MUSHROOMS

T (*testing for gluten—milkless, eggless, cornless*)

12–14 large fresh mushrooms
½ cup milkless margarine
¼ cup chopped shallots, or
   scallions
¼ cup Roquefort cheese
   (imported/sheep), crumbled

4 tablespoons fresh bread crumbs
   (wheat bread)
¼ teaspoon salt
⅛ teaspoon pepper

Wash and clean mushrooms. Remove stems and dice. In a small skillet, sauté mushroom stems and shallots or scallions in margarine. Stir in crumbled Roquefort cheese and bread crumbs. Fill mushroom caps with mixture and place in a greased baking dish. Bake at 350° for 15 minutes.

Serves 12–14

NACHOS

T (*testing for corn—eggless, glutenless*)

1 eight-ounce can refried beans
1 package wedge-shaped corn
    tortilla chips
9 ounces Cheddar cheese, grated
9 ounces Monterey Jack cheese,
    grated

¼ cup chopped green chiles
1 can (2½ ounces) ripe olives,
    sliced
Guacamole Dip*
Tomato wedges

On an ovenproof platter, place half of refried beans, patting them down. Place half of tortilla chips on top of refried beans. In a bowl, mix grated cheeses and green chiles. Sprinkle cheese mixture on top of chips. Repeat with beans, chips, and cheeses. Place under broiler (or in a microwave oven) until cheese melts. Garnish with ripe olives, guacamole dip, and tomato wedges. Serve hot.

Serves 6

SOUPS

BEEF STOCK

E (*milkless, eggless, glutenless, cornless*)

6 beef bones
½ pound inexpensive lean beef chuck
1 medium onion
1 medium carrot
1 celery stalk, including leaves
  Bouquet Garni*

3 cups water
1 large shallot, minced
  Freshly ground salt and pepper

Cut beef into 1-inch cubes. Cut carrot, onion, and celery into chunks. Put beef bones, chuck, and vegetables in a hot oven and bake at 425° for 30 minutes. Transfer to a large saucepan; add bouquet garni, water, salt, and pepper. Cover and simmer for 6 hours. Strain stock through a sieve lined with cheesecloth.

Makes 1½–2 cups

CHICKEN STOCK

E (*milkless, eggless, glutenless, cornless*)

1 pound chicken wings
1 pound chicken necks
1 teaspoon salt
½ teaspoon freshly ground black
  pepper
  Bouquet Garni*

3-4 shallots, chopped
1 large leek
3 cups water
1 medium carrot, diced
1 celery stalk, thinly sliced

Place chicken, leeks, celery, carrot, and shallots into a greased baking pan. Bake at 425° for 30 minutes. Transfer to a large saucepan. Add bouquet garni, water, salt, and pepper. Cover and simmer for 6 hours. Strain stock through a sieve lined with cheesecloth.

Makes 1½–2 cups

PREPARED MISO BOUILLON

E (*milkless, eggless, glutenless, cornless*)

2 cups water
3 tablespoons red miso
½ teaspoon tamari (traditional/ wheat-free)
¼ cup sliced shallots

In a small saucepan, heat water to boiling. Reduce heat and add miso a little at a time, then add tamari. Serve immediately.

Serves 4

NOTE: This is a good source of lacto baccillus if you cannot eat yoghurt.

RUSSIAN BORSCH

E (*milkless, eggless, glutenless, cornless*)

4 cups Beef Stock* or 32 ounces of canned beef broth diluted with 1 quart of water
2 tablespoons milkless margarine
2 large carrots, peeled and sliced
1 cup chopped celery
1 cup chopped onion
2 cups just-cooked potatoes, not soft

2 cups shredded red cabbage
3 beets, peeled and shredded
2 cups fresh tomato wedges
2 tablespoons salt
2 teaspoons pepper
1 teaspoon dried marjoram
1 sprig fresh parsley, chopped

Prepare stock or broth. In a large kettle or saucepan, melt margarine. Add carrots and cook 5 minutes alone. Next add celery and onions. Sauté until tender. Add beef stock, potatoes, red cabbage, tomatoes, marjoram, salt, and pepper. Bring to a boil. Cook for 20–25 minutes. Serve hot. Garnish with parsley.

Serves 8

BROWN CABBAGE SOUP

E (*milkless, eggless, glutenless, cornless*)

1 cube (½ cup or 4 ounces)
   milkless margarine
1½ pounds cabbage, shredded
1 garlic clove, minced
1 tablespoon sugar
4 cups Beef Stock*
1 teaspoon salt
⅛ teaspoon pepper
¼ teaspoon ground allspice
1 bunch parsley, finely chopped

Melt margarine in a large saucepan and add cabbage and garlic. Sauté cabbage, turning frequently for 5 minutes. Sprinkle sugar over cabbage and simmer for 30 minutes until cabbage is brown all over. Add beef stock, salt, pepper, and allspice. Cover. Simmer for 1 hour or until cabbage is tender. Sprinkle with parsley. Serve hot.

Serves 8

CARROT SOUP

(*eggless, glutenless, cornless*)

2 tablespoons margarine
6 carrots, peeled and finely
   chopped
¼ cup chopped shallots
¼ cup minced celery
1 tablespoon soy flour
1 cup water

1 teaspoon salt
2 cups milk, or milk substitute
   (see Appendix A)
¼ cup freshly chopped parsley

In a saucepan, melt margarine. Add carrots, shallots, and celery, and sauté. Add flour and blend with vegetables. Slowly add water and salt. Cover. Simmer for 8 minutes over low heat. Uncover, add milk, and cook until soup is heated thoroughly. Serve with sprinkled parsley.

Serves 6–8

CORN CHOWDER

T (*testing for corn—milkless, eggless*)

2 tablespoons milkless margarine
½ cup chopped onion
5 medium potatoes, peeled and cubed
2 cups water
½ cup potato flour
½ cup milk substitute (see Appendix A)

2 cans creamed corn
1 teaspoon salt
⅛ teaspoon paprika
2 tablespoons chopped pimento
2 tablespoons chopped fresh parsley

Melt margarine in a large saucepan. Add onion and sauté until tender. Add potatoes and water and cook until potatoes are done. In a separate bowl, mix potato flour and milk. Add this to cooked potatoes and mix well. Add creamed corn, salt, and paprika. Simmer for 10 minutes. Garnish with pimento and parsley.

Serves 4

CREAM OF CELERY SOUP

E (*milkless, eggless, glutenless, cornless*)

¼ cup milkless margarine
½ onion, finely chopped
1 cup finely chopped celery
1 cup potato pieces
1 cup Chicken Stock*
1½ teaspoons celery salt
1 bay leaf
1 teaspoon salt
¼ teaspoon white pepper

2 cups milk substitute (see Appendix A)
2 tablespoons parsley

In a saucepan, melt margarine. Add onion and celery and sauté until tender. Add potatoes, chicken stock, celery salt, bay leaf, salt, and pepper. Cook until potatoes are tender. Remove from heat. Put mixture into a blender or food processor and purée. Pour back into saucepan. Add milk substitute and heat thoroughly. Serve hot with parsley as garnish.

Serves 4–6

CREAM OF CHICKEN SOUP

E (*milkless, eggless, glutenless, cornless*)

½ onion, finely chopped
¼ cup milkless margarine
1 cup finely chopped celery
1 cup Chicken Stock*
½ cup chopped cooked chicken

1 teaspoon salt
¼ teaspoon pepper
1½ cups milk substitute (see Appendix A)

In a saucepan, melt margarine. Add onion and celery, and sauté until tender. Add remaining ingredients and cook until chicken is tender and soup is thick. Pour into a blender or food processor and purée. Return soup to saucepan, add milk substitute, and heat thoroughly.

Serves 4

CREAM OF TOMATO SOUP

E (*milkless, eggless, glutenless, cornless*)

2 cups soy milk
1 fifteen-ounce can tomatoes, finely chopped
2 tablespoons arrowroot flour or soy flour

½ cup finely chopped onion
1 teaspoon salt
½ teaspoon pepper

Heat milk in a saucepan. Using a whisk, whip in the rest of the ingredients. Bring to a boil, then lower heat and simmer for 15 minutes. Serve immediately.

Serves 4

EGGPLANT AND ONION SOUP

T (*testing for milk—eggless, glutenless, cornless*)

2 tablespoons margarine
½ cup chopped onion
2 small (Japanese) eggplants, or 1 small eggplant, cut into cubes
1½ cups Beef Stock*

2 tablespoons prepared miso (see Food Ingredient Glossary)
⅓ cup Parmesan cheese
⅛ teaspoon pepper
2 tablespoons minced parsley

Melt margarine in a saucepan. Add onion and eggplant and sauté. Add beef stock and bring to a boil. Reduce heat, add miso and Parmesan, and return to boil. Serve topped with pepper and parsley.

Serves 4

LEMON AND CHICKEN SOUP

T (*testing for citrus—milkless, glutenless, cornless*)

1 four-pound chicken (male)	5 eggs (cooler than room
water to cover chicken	temperature)
1 cup rice	Juice of 2 lemons

Prepare a chicken broth by boiling chicken (remove skin) with enough water to cover. Cook until meat falls off bones. Strain and collect 8 cups of broth. Add 1 cup of uncooked rice. Cook rice covered for 20 minutes. Remove from heat. In a separate mixing bowl, beat eggs until thick, then add lemon juice, beating constantly. Gradually add hot broth to egg mixture, stirring soup constantly so it will not curdle.

Serves 6

LENTIL SOUP

E (*milkless, eggless, glutenless, cornless*)

1 cup lentils, rinsed and drained	½ teaspoon thyme
4 cups water	½ teaspoon nutmeg
2 tablespoons milkless margarine	1 tablespoon minced parsley
½ cup chopped shallots	1 bunch fresh spinach, cleaned
½ cup thinly sliced carrots	and chopped
½ cup chopped celery	3 tablespoons Prepared Miso
1 garlic clove, minced	Boullion*
¼ cup water	

Combine lentils and water in a large kettle and soak overnight. Bring to a boil and simmer for 2 hours until quite thick.

Meanwhile, melt margarine in a skillet and sauté shallots, carrots, celery, and garlic until tender. Add water and allow to simmer for 10–15 minutes.

Stir in thyme, nutmeg, parsley, spinach, and miso. Simmer 5–10 minutes more. Combine with lentils and allow to heat thoroughly.

Serves 8

FRENCH ONION SOUP

E (*milkless, eggless, glutenless, cornless*)

2 tablespoons milkless margarine
2 onions, thinly sliced
1 can (10½ ounces) beef broth
½ cup water
1 tablespoon tamari (traditional/
  wheat-free)
½ teaspoon salt
⅛ teaspoon pepper

In a saucepan, melt margarine. Add onion and sauté until tender. Add remaining ingredients, and heat thoroughly. Serve hot.

Serves 4

POTATO AND ONION SOUP

T (*testing for milk—eggless, glutenless, cornless*)

4 medium potatoes, peeled and diced
1 medium onion, thinly sliced
2 cups Chicken Stock*
2 bay leaves
2 tablespoons Prepared Miso Bouillon*
½ cup grated cheddar cheese
⅛ teaspoon pepper
1 tablespoon minced parsley

Combine potatoes, onion, chicken stock, and bay leaves and bring to a boil. Cover and simmer for 1 hour. Add miso and stir in cheese. Add pepper and heat to boiling. Remove from heat and top with parsley.

Serves 4–6

POTATO-SPINACH SOUP

E (milkless, eggless, glutenless, cornless)

4 tablespoons milkless margarine
¼ cup chopped onion
¼ cup chopped celery
3 tablespoons arrowroot flour,
  or potato flour
1 quart water

2½ cups diced potatoes
2 tablespoons salt
1½ cups chopped fresh spinach
½ cup non-dairy creamer
  (cornless variety, see
  Appendix A under Milk)

Melt margarine in a large saucepan. Sauté onion and celery until tender.
Lower heat and blend in flour. Add water, potatoes, and salt. Bring to a
boil, cover and simmer about 30 minutes until potatoes are tender. Stir
occasionally. Add spinach. Cook uncovered for 2 minutes, then add non-
dairy creamer. Serve hot.

Serves 6

SPINACH SOUP

(milkless, glutenless, cornless)

2 tablespoons milkless margarine
1 ten-ounce package frozen
  chopped spinach, drained and
  dried
2 tablespoons potato flour
1 tablespoon tapioca flour
4 cups Chicken Stock*
⅛ teaspoon fennel seed
1 egg yolk
½ cup non-dairy creamer (cornless
  variety, see Appendix A under
  Milk)

Melt margarine in a saucepan. Add two flours slowly, then gradually add
chicken stock. Add chopped spinach, and cover and simmer for 20 minutes.
Season with fennel. In a separate small mixing bowl, blend egg yolk and
non-dairy creamer until smooth, and add to soup. Serve warm.

Serves 8

SPLIT PEA SOUP

T (*testing for pork—milkless, eggless, glutenless, cornless*)

1 pound (2 cups dried) split peas
2 quarts water
  Ham shank
½ cup chopped onion
1 cup chopped celery
1 sprig parsley
¼ teaspoon pepper
2 teaspoons salt
1 whole bay leaf

Follow instructions on bag for cooking split peas. After soaking peas, add ham, onion, celery, parsley, pepper, and salt. Cook for 4 hours.

Serves 6

COLD TOMATO AVOCADO SOUP

E (*milkless, eggless, glutenless, cornless*)

3 cups Cream of Tomato Soup*
1 ripe avocado, peeled and diced
1 garlic clove, minced
¼ teaspoon salt
⅛ teaspoon cayenne
⅛ teaspoon pepper
¼ cup non-dairy creamer (cornless
  variety, see Appendix A under
  Milk)
¼ cup sesame seeds
2 tablespoons freshly chopped
  parsley

Combine tomato soup, avocado, garlic, salt, pepper and cayenne. Purée this mixture in a blender or food processor. Serve with non-dairy creamer, sesame seeds, and parsley.

Serves 6

TOMATO AND CORN SOUP

T (*testing for corn—milkless, eggless, glutenless*)

2 tablespoons milkless margarine
2 tablespoons diced green pepper
1 cup thinly sliced onion
1 small can corn kernels
2 medium tomatoes, diced
1 cup milk substitute (see
    Appendix A)
2 tablespoons Prepared Miso
    Bouillon*
⅛ teaspoon pepper
¼ teaspoon oregano
2 tablespoons minced parsley

Melt margarine in a saucepan. Sauté green pepper, onion, and corn. Add tomatoes and sauté for 1 minute. Stir in milk substitute, miso, pepper, and oregano. Stir constantly. Do not let it boil. Cool. Pour into a blender or food processor and purée. Return to saucepan and heat thoroughly to just boiling. Serve hot with parsley on top.

Serves 4

NOTE: This soup can be prepared ahead to point where it is puréed, then reheated.

TURKEY RICE SOUP

E (*milkless, eggless, glutenless, cornless*)

3 cups chopped cooked turkey
1½ quarts water
1 tablespoon salt
2 tablespoons chopped parsley
½ teaspoon pepper
½ cup chopped celery
½ cup chopped carrots
½ cup rice
½ cup Chicken Stock*

Put all ingredients into a large saucepan. Simmer until rice, carrots, and celery are tender.

Serves 4

VEGETABLE SOUP I

E (*milkless, eggless, glutenless, cornless*)

1 cup Beef Stock*
1 fifteen-ounce can tomatoes, cut
   up with their liquid
½ cup sliced carrots
½ cup sliced celery
1 teaspoon salt
1 tablespoon Italian seasoning
   (see Ingredient Glossary under
   Herbs and Spices)
2 dashes pepper sauce

Mix all ingredients together. Cook until vegetables are tender. Serve hot.

Serves 4

VEGETABLE SOUP II

E (*milkless, eggless, glutenless, cornless*)

1 pound beef shank
¼ cup chopped onion
2 bay leaves
1½ quarts water
1 tablespoon salt
½ cup chopped celery
½ cup chopped carrots
½ cup chopped green pepper
½ cup chopped potatoes
5 peppercorns
1 tablespoon chopped parsley

Combine beef shank, onion, bay leaves, salt, peppercorns and water in a large saucepan. Simmer for 3 hours until meat is tender. Remove bones and peppercorns, and skim off fat. Add celery, carrots, green pepper, potatoes, and parsley to broth. Cover and cook 25 minutes, or until vegetables are tender.

Serves 6

VICHYSSOISE

E (*milkless, eggless, glutenless, cornless*)

4 large leeks, sliced
1 medium onion, sliced
2 tablespoons milkless margarine
¼ cup Chicken Stock*
3 cups boiling water
1¼ cups thinly sliced raw potatoes
1 cup milk substitute (see
   Appendix A)
¼ cup sliced shallots
Snipped chives
Salt and pepper to taste

Wash leeks, cut off their green tops, and slice white parts very thin. Melt margarine in a saucepan; add leeks and onion. Cover and cook over low heat for 10 minutes, but do not brown. Combine chicken stock and boiling water. Add leeks and onion, along with potatoes and pepper. Simmer until potatoes and leeks are done. Press through a seive or purée in blender or food processor. Cool. Add milk and chill for 3 hours. Garnish with chives. Salt and pepper to taste.

Serves 8

CHINESE VEGETABLE SOUP

E (*milkless, eggless, glutenless, cornless*)

2 tablespoons milkless margarine
¼ cup thinly sliced carrots
¼ cup raw green beans, cut into thin slivers
¼ cup thinly sliced water chestnuts
¼ cup minced celery
¼ cup chopped shallots

1 cup thinly sliced mushrooms
2 cups clear Chicken or Beef Stock*
1 tablespoon tamari (traditional/wheat-free)
1 cup chopped watercress

In a saucepan, melt margarine. Add carrots, green beans, water chestnuts, celery, shallots, and mushrooms. Sauté briefly. Add chicken or beef stock and tamari, and bring to a boil. Cook for 5 minutes. Add watercress and serve immediately.

Serves 4

ZUCCHINI SOUP

E (*milkless, eggless, glutenless, cornless*)

2 cups chopped zucchini
½ cup sliced shallots
1 cup finely chopped celery
¼ cup chopped parsley
2 teaspoons sweet basil
1 garlic clove, minced
2 medium potatoes, peeled and chopped

2 cans (10½ ounces) chicken broth or 2½ cups Chicken Stock*
½ teaspoon celery seasoning
⅛ teaspoon poultry seasoning
1 teaspoon salt
¼ teaspoon pepper
paprika

In a large saucepan, place zucchini, shallots, celery, parsley, basil, garlic, potatoes, broth or stock, and seasonings. Cover and simmer for 20–30 minutes or until zucchini and potatoes are tender. Let cool. Put in blender or food processor and purée until smooth. Reheat before serving and sprinkle with paprika.

Serves 6–8

FISH DISHES

COMPANY HALIBUT

E (*milkless, eggless, glutenless, cornless*)

1½ pounds fresh halibut
1 tablespoons milkless margarine
½ cup chopped onion
1 garlic clove, minced
¼ cup chopped green pepper
1 cup sliced celery
1 cup sliced carrots
2 sixteen-ounce cans tomatoes
1 cup Chicken Stock*
1 teaspoon salt
¼ teaspoon thyme
¼ teaspoon basil
¼ cup chopped fresh parsley

Cut halibut into 1-inch cubes. In a 10-inch skillet, melt margarine, add onion, garlic, green pepper, celery, and carrots, and sauté. Add tomatoes, chicken stock, salt, pepper, thyme, basil, and 2 tablespoons parsley. Cover and simmer for 25 minutes. Add halibut. Cover and simmer 15 minutes more. Sprinkle with remaining parsley.

Serves 4

HALIBUT WITH TOMATOES

E (*milkless, eggless, glutenless, cornless*)

2 tablespoons milkless margarine
¼ cup chopped onion
1 garlic clove, minced
1½ pounds fresh halibut steaks
2 small tomatoes, chopped
¼ cup Chicken Stock*
2 tablespoons chopped parsley
½ teaspoon salt
⅛ teaspoon white pepper
⅓ cup milk substitute (see
   Appendix A)
2 teaspoons tapioca flour

In a 10-inch skillet, sauté onion and garlic until tender. Add halibut, tomatoes, chicken stock, parsley, salt, and pepper. Cover and simmer over low heat until fish flakes easily when tested with a fork, about 10–12 minutes. In a small mixing bowl, combine milk and tapioca flour and add to skillet. Cook and stir until sauce is thickened and bubbly. Serve hot.

Serves 4

SALMON PATTIES

(*milkless, glutenless, cornless*)

1 can (15½ oz.) salmon
½ cup chopped onion
¼ cup chopped fresh parsley
1 cup fine dry rice bread* crumbs
1 beaten egg (or substitute, see
   Appendix A)
½ teaspoon poppy seeds
⅛ teaspoon dried tarragon
3 tablespoons oil

Drain and flake salmon, reserving ⅓ cup of liquid. In a large mixing bowl, combine salmon, onion, parsley, and bread crumbs. Add beaten egg (or substitute), poppy seeds, tarragon, and reserved salmon liquid. Shape into patties. In a large skillet, fry patties in oil until both sides are lightly brown.

Serves 4

TOMATOES WITH SALMON STEAKS

E (*milkless, eggless, glutenless, cornless*)

6 salmon steaks
2 tablespoons milkless margarine
½ cup finely chopped onion
1 pound canned tomatoes, finely
   chopped
4 tablespoons wine vinegar
2 drops Tabasco sauce
2 teaspoons salt
1 teaspoon white pepper

Place steaks in a large casserole dish. In a mixing bowl, mix onion, tomatoes, vinegar, Tabasco sauce, salt and pepper. Pour over steaks and marinate in refrigerator overnight. Place casserole dish in a moderate 375° oven and bake 30 minutes or until tender.

Serves 6

SALMON PIE

E (*milkless, eggless, glutenless, cornless*)

1 fifteen-ounce can salmon, packed in its own juices, washed and drained
1¼ cup cooked white rice
2 tablespoons chopped onion
1-2 pounds sliced fresh mushrooms (substitute 3 hard-boiled eggs when not on elimination diet)
2 teaspoons parsley
¼ cup milkless margarine
1 tablespoon potato flour
2 tablespoons tapioca flour
1 teaspoon curry powder
1 teaspoon salt
¼ teaspoon pepper
1 cup milk substitute (see Appendix A)

Melt margarine in a saucepan. Blend in tapioca and potato flour. Add salt, pepper, and curry powder. Add milk slowly until you have a smooth sauce. In a separate bowl, mix salmon, cooked rice, parsley, onion and 2 eggs, chopped (or mushrooms). Mix sauce and salmon mixture together. Pat into a greased 9-inch pie tin. Cover with 1 sliced hard-boiled egg. Cook covered 30 minutes at 350° or until hot.

Serves 8

BAKED BROCCOLI AND SOLE

E (*milkless, eggless, glutenless, cornless*)

1 bunch fresh broccoli, chopped and cooked, or 1 ten-ounce package frozen chopped broccoli
4 fresh sole fillets
½ cup sliced fresh mushrooms
1 cup Cream of Chicken Soup* or Cream of Celery Soup*

¼ cup freshly grated Romano cheese (imported/sheep)
½ teaspoon dill weed
½ teaspoon salt
¼ teaspoon pepper
¼ teaspoon ground nutmeg
1 tablespoon tamari (traditional/ wheat-free)

Place chopped broccoli in bottom of a foil-lined pan. Place fillets of sole over broccoli, and top fish with sliced mushrooms.

In a separate mixing bowl, combine soup, cheese, dill weed, salt, pepper, nutmeg, and tamari, and pour over fish. Close and seal foil. Bake at 350° for 1 hour or until fish is done.

Serves 4

SOLE WITH CAPERS

T (*testing for citrus—milkless, eggless, glutenless, cornless*)

3 tablespoons olive oil
1½ pounds fresh sole fillets
3 tablespoons potato flour
⅓ cup chopped fresh parsley
1½ tablespoons capers, drained and chopped
3 tablespoons rice bread* crumbs
1½ teaspoons lemon juice

Preheat oven to 425°. Put olive oil in a 10-inch skillet. Dip fish in flour, place in skillet over medium heat, and sauté until golden brown. Remove fish to a warm casserole dish. Add chopped parsley and capers to skillet with 1½ teaspoons of lemon juice and sauté 2 minutes. Add bread crumbs and stir. Spread bread crumb mixture over fillets. Bake fish in oven for 20 minutes or until fish flakes easily. Serve hot.

Serves 4

ROMANO SOLE

T (*testing for eggs—milkless, glutenless, cornless*)

1½ pounds fresh sole fillets
1 teaspoon salt
1 teaspoon dill weed
1 tablespoon chopped fresh
  parsley
½ cup Chicken Stock*
  Milk substitute (see
  Appendix A)

⅓ cup milkless margarine
2 tablespoons soy flour
5 eggs, separated (room
  temperature)
2 tablespoons freshly grated
  Romano cheese (imported/
  sheep)

Place fish in a 10 × 2-inch greased baking dish and sprinkle with salt, dill, and parsley. Pour chicken stock over fish, cover, and bake at 400° for 10 minutes. Drain off stock. Measure and add milk substitute to make 1 cup of liquid. Melt margarine, add flour, gradually stir in liquid, and cook until thickened. Remove from heat and beat in egg yolks. In a separate bowl, beat egg whites until stiff but not dry. Mix one-quarter of egg whites into stock. Fold in remaining egg whites. Sprinkle 1 tablespoon cheese over fish. Spoon sauce over fish and cheese, sprinkle with remaining cheese, and bake uncovered at 400° for 15 minutes.

Serves 4

BAKED SNAPPER AVOCADO BOATS

T (*testing for citrus—milkless, eggless, glutenless, cornless*)

3 tablespoons milkless
  margarine, melted
1 garlic clove, minced
2 tablespoons sliced onion
2 tablespoons chopped red
  pimento
1½ pounds red snapper

½ cup Chicken Stock*
3 ripe avocados
1 teaspoon salt
3 tablespoons lemon juice
½ cup cooked rice
¼ teaspoon paprika

In a large skillet, melt margarine. Add garlic, onion, and pimento. Sauté until tender. Add red snapper and chicken stock. Cover and simmer for 25 minutes. Meanwhile, cut avocados in half lengthwise, remove pits, and sprinkle them with lemon juice and salt. Drain cooked mixture and add to cooked rice and spices. Fill avocado boats with mixture, sprinkle with paprika and bake at 350° for 15 minutes.

Serves 6

SNAPPER IN FOIL

E (*milkless, eggless, glutenless, cornless*)

1½ pounds fresh snapper
1½ teaspoons tamari (traditional/
    wheat-free)
2 tablespoons freshly grated
    Romano cheese (imported/
    sheep)
1 cup Cream of Chicken Soup*
3 tablespoons grated onion
1 teaspoon basil
½ teaspoon salt
⅛ teaspoon pepper

Put some foil in bottom of an ovenproof casserole dish. Lay fish on top of foil, and sprinkle with cheese and tamari sauce. Pour on cream of chicken soup. Sprinkle with onion and spices. Cover with foil and fold air tight. Cook at 375° for 40 minutes until snapper is tender.

Serves 4

RED SNAPPER WITH GREEN PEPPER

E (*milkless, eggless, glutenless, cornless*)

1½ to 2 pounds snapper fillets
3 tablespoons olive oil
1 cup sliced onion
1 cup sliced green pepper
1 garlic clove, minced
½ cup fresh parsley, finely chopped
1 pound canned tomatoes, finely
    chopped
½ cup tomato sauce
Salt and pepper to taste

Prepare fillets. In a large skillet, heat olive oil until medium hot. Add fish and sauté until lightly brown on both sides. Remove and set aside. Add onions and green peppers and sauté until tender. Add garlic and sauté another minute. Stir in parsley, tomatoes, tomato sauce, salt, and pepper. Bring to a boil. Reduce heat, cover and simmer 10 minutes. Add fish and simmer 15 minutes more. Cool. Serve cold with bread.

Serves 4

NEW ORLEANS SNAPPER

E (*milkless, eggless, glutenless, cornless*)

½ cup milkless margarine
2 pounds fresh red snapper, cut into 1-inch cubes
¼ cup chopped onion
¼ cup chopped shallots
1 eight-ounce can tomatoes, cut up
1 clove garlic, minced
½ teaspoon thyme

½ teaspoon basil
2 tablespoons parsley flakes
1 cup Chicken Stock*
3 tablespoons arrowroot flour
Hot cooked rice

In a large skillet, melt the margarine and sauté onions, green pepper, and garlic. Add tomatoes with their juice, chicken stock, seasonings, and parsley. Add cubed fish. Simmer for 10–15 minutes until fish flakes. In a separate saucepan, prepare White Sauce II.* Add white sauce to fish mixture. Simmer and stir until sauce has thickened. Serve over rice.

Serves 4–6

FISH ROYALE

T (*testing for citrus—milkless, eggless, glutenless, cornless*)

2 pounds fresh or saltwater fish fillets
4 tablespoons lemon juice
1 tablespoon sea salt
½ teaspoon paprika
¼ teaspoon turmeric
¼ cup chopped onion
1 green pepper, cut into strips
2 fresh tomatoes, sliced

Marinate fish in a shallow dish with liquid made of lemon juice, salt, paprika, and turmeric, for at least 1 hour, turning the fish after 30 minutes.

In a saucepan, sauté onions in margarine until are just tender. Place onions, green pepper strips, and fresh tomato slices on top of fish fillets and bake for 20 minutes at 400°, or until fish flakes easily.

Serves 6

FISH SUPREME

E (*milkless, eggless, glutenless, cornless*)

1½ pounds fish fillets (snapper, bass, etc.)
1 teaspoon salt
4 fresh tomatoes, sliced
2 tablespoons milkless margarine
2 tablespoons sweet rice flour

½ cup milk substitute (see Appendix A)
1 teaspoon basil leaves
¼ cup Chicken Stock*
2 tablespoons minced parsley

Grease an 8 × 8 × 2-inch baking pan or ovenproof dish. Lay a single layer of fish in the pan. Sprinkle fish with half of the salt. Lay the sliced tomatoes over the fish, and sprinkle with the rest of the salt. Set baking pan aside.

In a saucepan, melt margarine. Add flour to margarine and blend. Slowly add milk substitute. Cook over low heat until slightly thick. Remove from heat and add basil and chicken stock. Pour sauce over fish and tomatoes. Sprinkle with parsley flakes, and bake in a 375° oven for 25 minutes, or until fish flakes easily with a fork.

Serves 4

TARRAGON OVEN-FRIED FISH

E (*milkless, eggless, glutenless, cornless*)

2 pounds fish fillets (sole, snapper, halibut)
½ teaspoon salt
1 cup dry rice bread* crumbs
1½ teaspoons tarragon

½ cup milk substitute (see Appendix A)
3 tablespoons milkless margarine, melted

Prepare fish. Cut into small serving pieces. In a small mixing bowl, combine bread crumbs, tarragon, and salt. In a separate small bowl, place milk. Dip fish into milk, then into crumb mixture. Place in greased 13 × 9-inch pan, and cover with remaining crumb mixture. Top with melted margarine. Place in preheated 425° oven, and bake for 15 minutes or until fish flakes easily with fork.

Serves 6–8

STUFFED TROUT I

T (*testing for gluten—milkless, eggless, cornless*)

1 large trout (2½ pounds) or
   3 small trout
1 teaspoon salt
4 tablespoons milkless margarine
¼ cup chopped green pepper
¼ cup chopped onion

1 cup mushrooms, sliced
¼ cup chopped celery
2 tablespoons chopped fresh
   parsley
2 cups wheat bread crumbs
Dash cayenne pepper
2 tablespoons milkless margarine

Slice fish right down belly from head to tail, cutting not quite all the way through. Wipe out the inside of the fish with a cloth crusted in salt. Remove head and tail. Snip out gills.

In a large saucepan, melt margarine. Sauté green peppers, onion, mushrooms, and celery for about 8 minutes or until tender. Add parsley and cook 5 minutes more. Mix in bread crumbs and cayenne. Remove from heat. Make a ¼-inch incision lengthwise from tail to head down one side of the trout. Put the filling into the fish. Brush the fish well with melted margarine. Roll fish in foil, and place in a shallow baking pan. Bake at 375° for 30–40 minutes.

Serves 4–6

STUFFED TROUT II

T (*testing for citrus—milkless, eggless, glutenless, cornless*)

1 1–2½ pound trout or 3 small
   trout
Salt
Lemon juice
1 carrot, chopped finely
1 apple, unpeeled, chopped
½ cup rice bread* crumbs

2 tablespoons very finely chopped
   onion
1 tablespoon minced parsley
1 tablespoon minced fresh dill
1 tablespoon sesame seeds
2 tablespoons Dijon-type mustard
3 tablespoons milkless margarine

Wash and clean fish. Remove head. Cut fish from head to tail but not quite all the way through. Sprinkle fish with salt and lemon juice. Set aside. Mix together carrots, apple, bread crumbs, onion, parsley, dill, and sesame seeds. Stuff mixture into fish and truss, using small skewers. Make a ¼-inch incision lengthwise from tail to head down one side of the trout. Place fish in a shallow pan, rub mustard generously all over, and dot with margarine. Bake at 375° for 1 hour.

Serves 6

TUNA CASSEROLE

(*milkless, cornless*)

1 seven-ounce can tuna
¼ cup chopped onion
½ package frozen peas
2 tablespoons parsley
¼ cup rice bread* crumbs
6 ounces cooked macaroni
  noodles (check ingredients)

1 two-ounce jar pimento, chopped
White Sauce:
1 tablespoon milkless margarine
1 tablespoon flour
1 cup Chicken Stock*
¼ teaspoon salt
⅛ teaspoon pepper

To make the white sauce, melt the margarine in a saucepan. Add the flour, stirring until smooth. Add the salt and pepper. Slowly add the chicken stock, and cook until thickened.

Combine all ingredients except for bread crumbs with white sauce. Top with bread crumbs, and bake at 350° for 30 minutes in a casserole dish.

Serves 4

TUNA FISH TOFU MOUSSE

E (*milkless, eggless, glutenless, cornless*)

2 envelopes unflavored gelatin
½ cup cold water
⅔ cup Chicken Stock*
1 seven-ounce can tuna
½ cup finely chopped celery
¼ cup chopped green pepper
⅓ cup Eggless Mayonnaise I*
  (or see Appendix A)

1 tablespoon tomato paste
1 cup mashed tofu
¼ teaspoon white pepper
½ teaspoon tamari (traditional/
  wheat-free)
Black olives, parsley, and
  pimento

Grease a 1½-quart mold. In a small bowl mix gelatin with cold water and let it sit over a saucepan of warm water to dissolve. Boil chicken stock and stir in softened gelatin.

In a large mixing bowl, mix tuna and softened gelatin and blend well. Stir in celery, green pepper, mayonnaise, tomato paste, tofu, pepper, and tamari. Pour into prepared mold and chill for 2 hours until firm.

To unmold, place mold in hot water for a minute. Unmold onto a plate. Garnish with parsley, black olives, and pimento.

Serves 6

TUNA PATTIES

E (*milkless, eggless, glutenless, cornless*)

1 seven-ounce can tuna
¼ cup chopped onion
½ cup dry rice bread* crumbs
1 egg substitute (see Appendix A)

¼ teaspoon dried tarragon
2 tablespoons finely chopped celery

Combine all the ingredients, shape into patties, and fry in oil until lightly brown on both sides.

Serves 4

TUNA MIX FOR SALAD AND SANDWICHES

E (*milkless, eggless, glutenless, cornless*)

1 seven-ounce can tuna, packed in water
½ cup Eggless Mayonnaise I* (or see Appendix A)
¼ cup chopped celery

2 tablespoons chopped onions, optional
2 tablespoons chopped green peppers
¼ teaspoon salt
⅛ teaspoon pepper

Mix all ingredients in a bowl. Place on lettuce or slices of rice bread.*

Serves 4

OVEN-BAKED FISH

E (*milkless, eggless, glutenless, cornless*)

½ cup milkless margarine
1 pound fish fillets

1 tablespoon arrowroot flour
2 tablespoons potato flour

Melt margarine in a 9 × 13-inch pan in a 400° oven. Dip fillets in combined flours, place in pan and spoon some of the margarine over the fish. Bake at 400° for 25 minutes or until fish flakes easily.

Serves 4

DEEP-FRIED FISH

T (*testing for corn—milkless, eggless, glutenless*)

6 fish (trout or other freshwater
  fish; do not use any fatty fish)
  Safflower oil, sesame seed oil
1 cup cornmeal

Heat 1-2 inches of oil in a deep frying pan until hot. Dip each fish into cornmeal, then fry in oil until tender.

Serves 6

MEAT DISHES

CHUCK ROAST STEW

E (*milkless, eggless, glutenless, cornless*)

2½ pounds chuck roast, cut into
    1-inch cubes
 3 potatoes, peeled and cut up
 1 carrot, peeled and cut up
 2 celery sticks with stalks,
    chopped
 1 garlic clove
 1 tablespoon tamari (traditional/
    wheat-free)
 1 twelve-ounce can beef broth
    or 1½ cups Beef Stock*
 1 eight-ounce can tomato sauce
 1 teaspoon sweet basil leaves
 1 teaspoon thyme
 1 tablespoon salt

Put ingredients into a large dutch oven and cook at 300° for 2 to 3½ hours.
Or put in a crock pot on low for 6–8 hours.

Serves 8

FARMER'S STEW

E (*milkless, eggless, glutenless, cornless*)

2 tablespoons milkless margarine
1 onion, chopped
2 pounds beef chuck, cut into cubes
1 teaspoon thyme
Fresh ground salt and pepper
6 carrots, peeled, washed, cut in half, then julienned

1 cup celery, scraped and sliced
Bouquet Garni*
4 cups Beef Stock* or beef broth
⅓ teaspoon cayenne pepper
1½ pounds potatoes, peeled and cut into chunks

In a large flameproof casserole dish, melt margarine. Add onion and sauté until tender. Add beef, thyme, salt, and pepper and cook 20 minutes, turning meat frequently. Add carrots and celery. Cook another 5 minutes. Add bouquet garni, beef stock or broth, pepper, and potatoes. Bring to a boil. Cook until meat and potatoes are done.

Serves 8

HUNGARIAN GOULASH

E (*milkless, eggless, glutenless, cornless*)

2 tablespoons olive or sesame seed oil
1½ pounds chuck pot roast, cut into 1-inch cubes
⅓ cup rice flour or potato flour
1 teaspoon salt
½ cup chopped onion
½ eight-ounce can tomato sauce
½ cup Beef Stock*
1 cup water

1 teaspoon paprika
1 bay leaf
1 tablespoon tamari (traditional/wheat-free)
½ cup non-dairy creamer (cornless) mixed with
3 tablespoons rice flour
Dash cayenne pepper (not during elimination diet)

In a large skillet with hot oil, brown chuck roast cubes after coating them with a mixture of flour and salt. Drain excess oil. Add onion, tomato sauce, beef stock, water, paprika, and bay leaf. Cover and simmer 1–1¾ hours until beef is tender. Add tamari, and then add mixture of non-dairy creamer and flour. Add a dash of cayenne. Do not cook for more than 15 minutes after adding creamer. Serve on rice during elimination diet.

Serves 6

BASIC MEAT LOAF

(milkless, glutenless, cornless)

1 pound ground sirloin or chuck
2 eggs (or egg substitute, see
  Appendix A)
½ cup rice bread* crumbs
⅓ cup tomato juice
½ cup chopped onion
¼ cup chopped green pepper
1 teaspoon salt
¼ teaspoon garlic salt
1 teaspoon prepared miso
1 eight-ounce can tomato sauce

Combine above ingredients in a large bowl and turn mixture into a shallow baking pan. Bake at 350° for 1 hour. Drain off any excess grease. Pour tomato sauce over meat loaf and bake for 10 minutes more.

Serves 4

BUCKWHEAT LOAF

T *(testing for eggs—milkless, glutenless, cornless)*

1 pound ground beef
1 cup cooked buckwheat
½ cup shredded carrots
¼ cup chopped parsley
½ cup chopped onion
½ cup chopped green pepper
¼ teaspoon powdered garlic
2 eggs
1 two-ounce jar pimento, chopped,
  with liquid

Mix all ingredients together and form a small mound. Mix a small amount of catsup and mustard together. Spread mixture over meat loaf mound. Bake in a 8 × 8 × 2-inch pan at 350° for 1 hour.

Serves 4

SESAME SEED MEAT LOAF

(*milkless, glutenless, cornless*)

1 pound lean ground beef
½ cup rice bread* crumbs
¼ cup crushed rice snap crackers
1 egg, beaten
¼ cup sesame seeds
¼ cup chopped onions
¼ cup chopped green pepper
3 tablespoons prepared miso
1 teaspoon garlic powder
¼ cup water or milk substitute (see
    Appendix A)

Mix all ingredients together and mold into a half-ball. Place in a 8 × 8 × 2-inch greased casserole dish. Top with homemade tomato sauce and mustard. Bake in 350° oven for 1 hour.

Serves 4

BARBECUE BEANS

E (*milkless, eggless, glutenless, cornless*)

1 pound pinto beans
1 quart water
2 tablespoons vegetable oil
2 onions, peeled and chopped
2–4 small green peppers, seeded and
    chopped
2 garlic cloves, peeled and crushed
1 pound ground beef

½ teaspoon rosemary
½ teaspoon oregano
2 teaspoons chili powder
2 teaspoons salt
2 tablespoons sugar
¼ teaspoon pepper
1 can (1 lb. 3 oz.) tomatoes

Wash and pick over beans, and place them in a large kettle with water. Cover and bring to a boil. Boil gently for 10 minutes. Remove beans from heat and let stand 1 hour. Meanwhile, in a large skillet, sauté onion, peppers, and garlic in vegetable oil until tender. Add beef and brown. Drain excess oil. Add meat mixture to beans, stirring well. Add remaining ingredients. Cover and simmer until beans are tender, about 3 hours.

Serves 8–10

BEEF ENCHILADAS

T (*testing for corn—eggless, glutenless*)

Filling:
1 pound Cheddar cheese (sharp)
1 pound Monterey Jack cheese
1 small can chopped olives
1 pound lean ground beef
½ cup chopped onions
1 garlic clove, minced
1 eight-ounce can tomato sauce

24 corn tortillas
½–1 cup oil

Sauce:
1 sixteen-ounce can tomato sauce
½–1 teaspoon chili powder
Salt (pinch)
Pepper (pinch)
½ can water

Grate cheeses and combine with olives in a medium-size bowl. Set aside. In a 10-inch skillet, brown meat, and then drain off grease. Add onions and garlic and sauté until tender. Mix in tomato sauce, salt, and pepper. Simmer for 10 minutes.

Meanwhile, in a small skillet fry each tortilla in 1 inch of oil on both sides for just a few seconds. Pat oil out of each tortilla and put at the beginning of an assembly line for enchiladas. On each tortilla place 2 tablespoons of meat mixture, then 2 tablespoons of cheese mixture. Roll, secure with a toothpick (if needed), and place rolled enchiladas side by side in an ungreased 9 × 13-inch baking pan. Bake at 350° for 30 minutes or until cheese melts.

While enchiladas are cooking, in a separate saucepan place tomato sauce, chili powder, salt, and water (from swished-out tomato can). Simmer until somewhat thick. Pour sauce over enchiladas and serve.

Serves 6–8

NOTE: You can substitute goat Cheddar and Jack for cow Cheddar and Jack.

EASY HAMBURGER AND RICE

(*milkless, eggless, glutenless*)

1 pound ground beef
1 cup cooked rice
1 cup catsup (contains corn syrup)
½ cup water

½ cup chopped onion
½ teaspoon salt
Pepper to taste

Brown ground beef and onion together; drain off any grease. Add catsup, water, and rice, and season with salt and pepper. Simmer 15 minutes.

Variations: Add mushrooms or green peppers.

Serves 4

SALISBURY STEAK

(*eggless, glutenless*)

1½ pounds lean ground chuck
½ cup chopped onion
½ teaspoon salt
½ teaspoon Italian seasoning (see Ingredient Glossary under *Herbs and Spices*)
¼ teaspoon turmeric
¼ teaspoon paprika
1 teaspoon onion salt
1 teaspoon garlic salt
⅛ teaspoon pepper
2 tablespoons oil

Sauce:
½ pound mushrooms, sliced
2 tablespoons margarine (optional)
3 tablespoons arrowroot flour
½ cup Beef Stock*
½ teaspoon Worcestershire sauce
¼ cup milk (or substitute, see Appendix A)

Combine beef, onion, and seasonings; pat mixture into 4 oval-shaped forms. Cook Salisbury steaks in a saucepan in oil until done to taste. Remove steaks from saucepan and keep warm. Add mushrooms and margarine to saucepan and sauté until done. Put mushrooms to side of pan; add arrowroot flour (add more margarine if necessary); stir until smooth. Slowly add stock and milk. Season with Worcestershire sauce. Allow mixture to thicken, pour over rice, and serve with steaks.

Serves 6

SWEET-SOUR MEATBALLS

(milkless, glutenless, cornless)

2 slices rice bread*
½ cup milk substitute (see
    Appendix A)
1½ pounds ground beef
2 eggs, beaten (or substitute, see
    Appendix A)
¼ cup chopped onion
½ teaspoon salt

⅛ teaspoon pepper
    Tapioca flour
¼ cup safflower oil
½ cup sliced shallots
1 eight-ounce can tomato sauce
1 cup Beef Stock*
2 tablespoons vinegar
⅓ cup brown sugar
⅓ cup raisins or currants

Soak rice bread in milk substitute. In a large mixing bowl, add soaked bread, beef, eggs, onion, salt, and pepper. Mix well. Form mixture into balls, then roll them in tapioca flour. In a large skillet add onions and oil, and sauté until tender. Add meatballs, and cook until browned on all sides. Add tomato sauce, beef stock, vinegar, sugar, and currants. Add salt and pepper to taste. Cover and simmer 40 minutes or until meatballs are done. Stir periodically so the meatballs will not stick.

Serves 6

STUFFED GREEN PEPPERS

E *(milkless, eggless, glutenless, cornless)*

1 pound ground beef
½ cup diced onion
1 teaspoon Italian seasoning (see
    Ingredient Glossary under
    Herbs and Spices)

1 sixteen-ounce can tomato sauce
1½ cups cooked rice
4 green peppers

Preheat oven to 400°. Brown ground beef and onion together. Add tomato sauce and seasoning and simmer for 15 minutes. Add cooked rice to mixture. Cut tops off each pepper; remove seeds and membrane. Blanch peppers in boiling water and rinse with cold water. Spoon beef-and-onion mixture into each pepper. Place stuffed peppers in greased caserole dish. Bake in oven for 15 minutes or until peppers are thoroughly heated.

Serves 4

BEEF SAUSAGES

E (*milkless, eggless, glutenless, cornless*)

2 pounds lean ground beef
1 garlic clove, minced
½ teaspoon allspice
½ teaspoon thyme

1¼ teaspoons salt
½ cup Beef Stock*
⅛ teaspoon white pepper
4 tablespoons safflower oil

Blend all ingredients together except for stock and oil. Beat in stock until mixture is smooth and fluffy. Divide into 20 sections, and roll each section into lengths approximately 3 inches long and 1 inch wide. Heat oil in a large skillet. Fry each sausage until crisp and brown.

Serves 20

DAVE'S SPAGHETTI MEAT SAUCE

E (*milkless, eggless, glutenless, cornless*)

2 tablespoons olive oil
1 pound ground beef
2 sixteen-ounce cans tomato sauce
1 six-ounce can tomato paste,
  mixed with 1 can of water
1 medium onion, diced
¼ pound fresh mushrooms, sliced

1 garlic clove, minced
1 tablespoon sugar
3 tablespoons Italian seasoning
  (see Ingredient Glossary under
  Herbs and Spices)
1 teaspoon oregano

Heat oil in a large skillet and brown ground beef. Drain off grease. Add mushrooms and onions, and sauté until onions are soft. Add remaining ingredients. Cover and simmer for 1½ to 2 hours.

Serves 4

NOTE: While on the elimination diet, serve over cooked spaghetti squash.

EASY CHILI

E (*milkless, eggless, glutenless, cornless*)

1 pound ground beef
1 medium onion, chopped
1 eight-ounce can tomato sauce
⅓ cup milk substitute (see
  Appendix A) or Cream of
  Tomato Soup*

1 tablespoon chili powder
1 sixteen-ounce can kidney beans

Sauté beef and onion in a large skillet. Drain excess oil. Add tomato sauce and milk substitute (or tomato soup), chili powder, and kidney beans. Simmer for 45 minutes to 1 hour.

Serves 4

MINCED MEATBALLS

(*milkless, glutenless, cornless*)

2 slices of day-old rice bread
1 cup milk substitute (see Appendix A)
1 pound lean ground beef
1 egg (or substitute, see Appendix A)
½ teaspoon salt
⅛ teaspoon white pepper

4 tablespoons freshly grated Romano cheese (imported/ sheep)
4 tablespoons freshly chopped parsley
1 tablespoon wine vinegar
¼ cup potato flour
2–3 tablespoons olive oil

Soften bread in milk. In a large mixing bowl, combine beef, egg, salt, pepper, cheese, parsley, and vinegar. Mix and knead mixture to make a paste. Form balls and roll them in flour. Fry meatballs in hot olive oil until golden.

Serves 4

EGGPLANT AND BEEF

E (*milkless, eggless, glutenless, cornless*)

4 tablespoons milkless margarine
½ cup sliced celery
½ cup chopped onion
¼ cup chopped green pepper
1 small eggplant, peeled and cubed
2 cups cooked beef

1 eight-ounce can tomato sauce and ¼ cup water
½ teaspoon salt
¼ teaspoon dried marjoram
⅛ teaspoon lemon pepper
⅛ teaspoon ground nutmeg
Dash allspice

Melt margarine in a large skillet. Sauté celery, onion, and green pepper until tender. Drain off excess margarine. Add eggplant, cooked beef, tomato sauce, water, salt, marjoram, pepper, nutmeg, and allspice. Cover and simmer for 45 minutes.

Serves 8

LILIAN'S BEEF JERKY

E (*milkless, eggless, glutenless, cornless*)

1½ pounds lean steak, roast, or
    other cut of beef
1 garlic clove, peeled
    Ground pepper
½ teaspoon salt

Marinade:
Combine in a mixing bowl
2 tablespoons miso
2 teaspoons tamari (traditional/
    wheat-free)
3 tablespoons brown sugar
½ cup safflower oil
2 tablespoons vinegar

Alternative Marinade:
    Beef Stock*

In a large casserole, marinate steak for 24 hours after rubbing it with garlic clove. Pat dry. Trim off fat. Cut strips from meat ⅛ inch or less in thickness. Cross-grain slices will be more tender than with-grain strips. Add salt and pepper to strips.

Place strips on rack of a baking pan. Bake in a preheated 150° oven for 4 hours. Prop oven door open at top approximately 3–6 inches. Turn strips several times during drying process. Test for dryness. Store in covered jars in a cool, dry place in refrigerator.

Makes approximately 25 pieces

MARINATED FLANK STEAK

E (*milkless, eggless, glutenless, cornless*)

1½ pound flank steak

Marinade:
  2 teaspoons tamari (traditional/
    wheat-free)
  2 tablespoons miso

3 tablespoons brown sugar
2 tablespoons vinegar
1 garlic clove, minced
½ cup safflower oil
2 shallots, sliced
1 teaspoon ground ginger

In a mixing bowl, combine marinade ingredients. Pour over steak. Marinate overnight in refrigerator. When ready to cook, pat meat dry and place on a cooking sheet. Place under broiler for 3–5 minutes. Slice diagonally and serve.

Serves 4–6

ORIENTAL PEPPER STEAK

E (*milkless, eggless, glutenless, cornless*)

1½ pounds round steak
3 tablespoons safflower oil
1 cup sliced onion
1 pound canned tomatoes
1 teaspoon salt
½ teaspoon white pepper
2 bay leaves
2 large green peppers, seeded and
  cut into strips
1 tablespoon tapioca flour

2 teaspoons tamari (traditional/
  wheat-free)
¼ cup cold water

Cut round steak into ¼-inch-wide strips. In a large skillet, heat oil, and brown meat strips quickly on both sides. Remove from skillet and set aside. Add onions and sauté until tender. Add tomatoes with liquid, salt, pepper, and bay leaves. Cover and simmer for 45 minutes to 1 hour. Stir in green peppers. Continue cooking 15 minutes longer.

In a separate mixing bowl, blend tapioca, tamari, and cold water, and add mixture to skillet. Cook until thickened, about 1 minute. Serve over a bed of rice.

Serves 4–6

EASY PINWHEEL FRANK CASSEROLE

(*eggless, glutenless*)

3 cups cooked rice
1 pound all-beef kosher frankfurters, sliced (leave 2 unsliced,
for topping)

1 twelve-ounce can whole kernel
corn
10 ounces Cream of Celery Soup*
thickened with tapioca flour
1 cup shredded Cheddar cheese

Preheat oven to 350°.

Place cooked rice in a 2-quart greased casserole. In a separate mixing bowl, combine sliced frankfurters, corn, cream of celery soup, and three-quarters of cheddar cheese. Place this mixture on top of rice. Cut remaining 2 frankfurters in half lengthwise, then in half crosswise. Place on top of casserole in a pinwheel design. Top with remaining cheese. Bake 20–30 minutes.

VARIATIONS: Use frozen green peas or lima beans in place of corn.

Serves 6

BASIC LAMB STEW

E (*milkless, eggless, glutenless, cornless*)

2 tablespoons oil
½ cup chopped onion
2½ pounds lamb, cut into 1-inch
cubes

1 cup water or Beef Stock*
2 cups chopped tomatoes
2 cups sliced potatoes
Salt and pepper

Heat oil in a large skillet. Sauté onions until tender. Add lamb and stock. Cover and simmer for 1 hour. Add tomatoes, potatoes, salt and pepper. Cover and simmer for 45 minutes.

Serves 8

BAKED LAMB CHOPS

T (*testing for milk—eggless, glutenless, cornless*)

4–6 thick lamb chops
1 cup sour cream
2 tablespoons rice flour

1 cup French Onion Soup*
thickened with tapioca flour
2 tablespoons minced parsley

In a 9 × 13-inch casserole dish or baking pan, place lamb chops under a *hot* broiler and brown for 8–10 minutes on each side (depending on thickness). In a mixing bowl, combine flour and sour cream. Add French onion soup and parsley. Pour mixture over lamb chops and cover. Bake at 350° for 1 hour.

Serves 4

LAMB CHOPS WITH TARRAGON

E (*milkless, eggless, glutenless, cornless*)

4 lamb chops
½ cup carrots, peeled
½ garlic clove, peeled
4 tablespoons milkless margarine
1 cup chopped onion

¼ teaspoon tarragon wine vinegar
½ cup chopped celery
½ cup Beef Stock*
1 teaspoon tarragon
Salt and pepper

Rub lamb chops with garlic clove. In a skillet, melt margarine and add onion, carrot, celery, and sauté until tender. Push vegetables to one side, add lamb chops, and season with salt and pepper. Sear lamb chops on both sides until meat is pink. Reduce heat. Drain off excess oil. Add beef stock, vinegar, and tarragon. Bring to a boil, reduce heat, cover and simmer until lamb is done.

Serves 4

LAMB CHOPS AND BEEF SAUSAGES WITH TOMATOES

E (*milkless, eggless, glutenless, cornless*)

¼ cup olive oil
8 lamb chops
Salt
Freshly ground pepper
Beef Sausages*
½ cup chopped onion
1 garlic clove, minced

1 sixteen-ounce can tomatoes, drained and chopped
1 bay leaf, crumbled
½ teaspoon thyme
½ cup water
¼ cup finely chopped fresh parsley

NOTE: You are using 2 skillets in this recipe.

In a large skillet, heat olive oil over medium high heat. Sprinkle chops with salt and ground pepper, and brown in oil quickly without burning until they are pink inside. Arrange chops in a 9 × 13-inch baking dish and set aside.

In a small skillet, place uncooked beef sausages. Add water to cover and boil for 3 minutes. Lower heat, cover and simmer for 5 minutes. Drain on paper towels. Slice sausages into 1-inch pieces and place over chops.

Add onion and garlic to skillet in which lamb was browned and sauté for 5 minutes or until tender. Add tomatoes, bay leaf, thyme, and water. Bring to a boil and cook for 5 minutes. Pour mixture over sausage and lamb chops. Cover and bake at 375° for 20 minutes. Uncover and bake 10 minutes more. Sprinkle with parsley and serve.

Serves 6

CARROT LAMB LOAF

T (*testing for eggs—milkless, glutenless, cornless*)

1½ pounds ground lamb
¼ cup chopped onion
2 cups grated carrots
1½ cups soft rice bread* crumbs
1 egg, beaten
½ cup tomato sauce
½ teaspoon tamari (traditional/
   wheat-free)
1 teaspoon salt
¼ teaspoon pepper
3 tablespoons chopped fresh
   parsley

Combine all ingredients and mix well. Press into a loaf pan. Bake at 350° for 1 hour. Pour off drippings.

Serves 6

LAMB AND BEANS

E (*milkless, eggless, glutenless, cornless*)

1 pound dried white beans
4 cups water
2 tablespoons safflower oil
1 cup chopped onion
1 garlic clove, minced
1 pound lean lamb, coarsely
 ground
1 sixteen-ounce can tomatoes
1 teaspoon salt
¼ cup minced parsley
½ teaspoon thyme

Soak beans overnight; drain. Add 4 cups of boiling water to beans. Let
stand 10 minutes. Drain again. In a large dutch oven or casserole, add oil,
onion, and garlic. Sauté until tender. Add lamb, tomatoes, salt, parsley,
and thyme. Simmer covered, for about 2½ hours. Serve hot.

Serves 4

EASY LAMB CASSEROLE

E (*milkless, eggless, glutenless, cornless*)

1 pound lamb shoulder, cut into
 1-inch cubes
1 cup uncooked rice
1 sixteen-ounce can tomato sauce
3 tablespoons safflower oil
1 clove garlic, minced
1 teaspoon salt
½ teaspoon dill weed
⅛ teaspoon pepper
3 large mushrooms, sliced
½ cup chopped green pepper
 (optional)

In a pan greased with oil, brown lamb until pink. Add seasonings, tomato
sauce, and rice. Bake for 30 minutes at 350° in a covered baking pan.

Serves 4–6

LAMB CURRY

E (*milkless, eggless, glutenless, cornless*)

2 tablespoons milkless
   margarine
1½ pounds diced shoulder of lamb
1 cup Beef Stock*
½ cup chopped onion

½ cup chopped celery
1 cup rice bread* crumbs
¼ teaspoon pepper
1½ teaspoons curry powder

In a 10-inch skillet, melt margarine. Add lamb and cook until pink. In a separate bowl, mix the rest of the ingredients, then pour over lamb. Cover and simmer for 1 hour, stirring occasionally.

Serves 4

LAMB AND EGGPLANT

E (*milkless, eggless, glutenless, cornless*)

1½ pounds coarsely ground lamb
½ cup chopped onion
½ cup pine nuts
¼ teaspoon pepper
¼ teaspoon salt
   Dash allspice
2–3 large eggplants, peeled and
   sliced
2–4 tablespoons olive oil

1 sixteen-ounce can tomato
   sauce
1 cup water
   Pinch of Dried Mint*

In a large skillet, sauté meat. Add onion, pine nuts, pepper, salt, and allspice. Remove mixture and set aside. Brush eggplant slices with oil and cook in skillet until lightly brown on both sides (you may need to add more oil since eggplant will absorb it). Arrange browned eggplant slices in a greased 9 × 13-inch baking pan. Place some meat mixture on top of each eggplant slice. Then place a slice of browned eggplant on top of meat mixture. Make a sauce of tomato sauce, water, and dried mint. Let this simmer 5 minutes, then pour it over casserole dish and bake in a 400° oven for 30 minutes.

Serves 6

LAMB KABOB

E (*milkless, eggless, glutenless, cornless*)

1 pound lamb, boneless
shoulder, cut into ½-inch cubes
2 tablespoons milkless
margarine
1½ cups Beef Stock*
1 tablespoon tamari (traditional/
wheat-free)

1 teaspoon salt
½ teaspoon pepper
Cut vegetables: canned whole
onions, whole mushrooms, cut
tomatoes, cut green peppers

Preheat frying pan to medium for vegetables; to medium high for lamb. Place vegetables (except tomatoes and onions) in a frying pan with ½ cup of the beef stock. Cook quickly over medium heat. Add tomatoes and onions; remove to a warm platter before the vegetables are tender. Increase heat of frying pan to medium high and add milkless margarine. (Your heat is too high if it starts smoking.) Add cubed lamb, seasoned with salt and pepper, and cook, stirring occasionally, until lamb is just pink. Remove to a warm platter. Decrease heat of frying pan to medium and add remaining beef stock and tamari. Scrape up the lamb drippings with the added liquid to make a sauce. Assemble kabobs, and lay them over a bed of rice. Pour sauce over all.

Serves 4

LAMB AND LIMA BEANS

E (*milkless, eggless, glutenless, cornless*)

6 tablespoons milkless
margarine
1-2 pounds lamb shoulder, cut
into 1-inch cubes
4 small onions, sliced
2 packages frozen lima beans
½ cup sliced mushrooms
6 fresh tomatoes (or 1 sixteen-
ounce can tomatoes)
½ cup water
Salt and pepper

In a skillet, melt 4 tablespoons of margarine over high heat. (If the margarine is smoking, your heat is too high.) Quickly sear lamb meat until brown and meat is just pink. Remove lamb; set aside. Melt remaining margarine with lamb drippings, and add onions and mushrooms; sauté until tender. Add lima beans, tomatoes, water, salt and pepper. Simmer until thickened. Return lamb to mixture and cook until meat is heated through, approximately 15 minutes. Serve over rice.

Serves 4–6

LAMB STUFFED IN GRAPE LEAVES

E (*milkless, eggless, glutenless, cornless*)

2 breasts of lamb (optional)
½ pound coarsely ground lamb
1 cup uncooked rice
2 tablespoons mint leaves
1 egg substitute (see Appendix
   A)
2 tablespoons chopped parsley
1 teaspoon salt
   Canned grape leaves
   Salt
1 fifteen-ounce can beef broth
1 eight-ounce can tomato sauce

Place both breasts of lamb on bottom of a dutch oven. Combine ground lamb, rice, mint leaves, egg, parsley, and salt. Wash grape leaves, and cut them into halves. Spoon 2 tablespoons of lamb mixture onto each grape leaf. Fold over sides of leaves and roll up, putting salt in between each layer. Place them in dutch oven. On top of leaves place an inverted oven-proof pan or casserole dish, that is smaller than the dutch oven, leaving space between it and the rim of the dutch oven. Pour beef broth into dish just to the level of the edge of the pan or casserole dish. At this point the liquid should just be covering the rolls of grape leaves. Bake at 350° for 30–40 minutes, or until the liquid bakes down. Add tomato sauce and cook for 5 more minutes.

Serves 4–6

MOUSSAKA

(milkless, glutenless, cornless)

Olive oil
1 large eggplant, peeled and cut into ½-inch slices
3 medium potatoes, peeled and cut into ¼-inch slices
3 medium zucchini, peeled and cut into ¼-inch slices
1½ pounds ground lamb or beef
1 clove garlic, chopped
1 cup chopped onions
½ cup sliced mushrooms

1½ teaspoons salt
1 eight-ounce can tomatoes, drained
1 eight-ounce can tomato sauce
3 tablespoons chopped fresh parsley
1½ teaspoons oregano
1 cup Béchamel Sauce*
3 eggs, beaten
⅓ cup freshly grated Romano cheese (imported/sheep)

In a large skillet, fry potato slices, then the zucchini and finally the eggplant until almost done, adding oil as needed. Set cooked vegetables aside. Drain off excess oil. Sauté meat, garlic, onions, and mushrooms until meat is brown. Pour off excess oil. Stir in tomatoes, tomato sauce, parsley, and oregano. Cover and simmer. Cook until liquid has reduced. Meanwhile, prepare Béchamel sauce.

Put half of the eggplant, potato and zucchini slices in a greased 9 × 13-inch baking dish. Spread meat mixture over and top with remaining vegetables. Add beaten eggs to cooled Béchamel sauce. Pour over layered mixture, and sprinkle with Romano. Bake in a 350° oven 35–45 minutes or until bubbly.

Serves 8

SFEEHA

(Syrian Meat Pie)
(milkless, eggless, cornless)

Dough:
1 package yeast
¾ cup warm water
½ teaspoon sugar
1 teaspoon salt
¼ cup safflower oil
2 cups sifted flour

Meat Filling:
2 pounds coarsely ground lamb
1 large onion, grated
Juice of 2 lemons
½ cup pine nuts

Dissolve yeast in warm water. Add sugar, salt, and oil. Stir in sifted flour. Dough should be soft. Lift onto a lightly floured pastry cloth. Coat fingers and hands with oil and knead 12–15 minutes. Put dough in a bowl, cover, and let stand in a warm place until double in size. While dough is rising, prepare meat mixture.

In medium-size bowl, mix together lamb, grated onion, and pine nuts.

When dough is ready, punch down, and place on a lightly floured pastry cloth. Divide into 12 pieces. Roll each piece in your hands to shape into balls. Roll out each ball into a circle. Place a small amount of meat mixture on top. Fold dough into triangles. Arrange meat pies on an oiled baking pan and bake at 450° for 15 minutes or until done.

Makes 12 pies

STUFFED CABBAGE ROLLS

E (*milkless, eggless, glutenless, cornless*)

¾ cup uncooked rice, rinsed in cold water	1 head cabbage, boiled until just limp
1½ pounds coarsely ground lamb	2 cloves garlic, chopped
½ teaspoon salt	1 sixteen-ounce can whole tomatoes, chopped
⅛ teaspoon pepper	Water, if needed
Dash of allspice and nutmeg	

In a medium-size bowl, mix rice, ground lamb, salt, pepper, allspice, and nutmeg. Place a small amount of meat mixture on each cooked cabbage leaf and roll. Place rolls in a dutch oven. Sprinkle chopped garlic in between rolls. Pour tomatoes with juice over cabbage rolls, adding enough water, if needed, to almost cover them. Bake at 350° for 20 minutes.

Serves 6

PASOLE

T (*testing for pork—milkless, eggless, glutenless*)

2 pounds pork chops or steaks	1 four-ounce can green chiles, diced
1 large can (32 ounces) hominy, with liquid	½ head shredded lettuce
1 large onion, diced	2 medium tomatoes, diced
1 tablespoon chili powder	

In a large skillet, brown meat with onions; drain. Place in an adequately sized pan and add hominy, chili powder, and chilies. Cover and cook over low heat for 1½–2 hours. Place on a platter. Garnish with shredded lettuce and tomatoes.

NOTE: This recipe has corn in it (hominy).

Serves 4

ROMANO HAM AND RICE

T *(testing for pork—milkless, eggless, glutenless, cornless)*

2 tablespoons milkless margarine	2 tablespoons minced parsley
½ cup chopped onion	Dash cayenne
1 cup sliced mushrooms	1 cup frozen peas
⅓ cup uncooked long-grain rice	½ teaspoon salt
1½ cups diced cooked ham	⅛ teaspoon pepper
1 cup Chicken Stock*	¼ cup grated Romano cheese (imported/sheep)

Melt margarine in a large skillet. Add onions and mushrooms and sauté until tender. Add rice, and sauté. Blend in ham, chicken stock, dash of cayenne, and parsley. Bring mixture to a boil. Pour into a 1-quart casserole. Cover and bake at 350° for 30 minutes. Remove casserole from oven. Add peas, salt, and pepper. Sprinkle Romano cheese over top, and bake an extra 15 minutes, uncovered.

Serves 4

POULTRY DISHES

BAKED CHICKEN TARRAGON

E (*milkless, eggless, glutenless, cornless*)

1 frying chicken (about 2½ pounds), skin removed
1 cup Chicken Stock*
½ cup milkless margarine
1 clove garlic, pressed
1 teaspoon paprika
1 green pepper, cut into strips
¼ cup chopped scallions
¼ pound mushrooms, sliced
1 teaspoon tarragon
2 tomatoes, cut into wedges
1 teaspoon salt

In ¼ cup of margarine, brown chicken on both sides with garlic and paprika. Remove chicken from pan, add remaining margarine, and sauté mushrooms, onions, and green pepper. Return chicken to pan. Add chicken stock, tarragon, tomatoes, and salt. Simmer for 1 hour or until chicken is tender. Serve over rice.

Serves 4

BRUNSWICK STEW

T (*testing for pork—milkless, eggless, glutenless*)

1 frying chicken, cut up
½ cup cooked ham, cubed
2 drops hot pepper sauce
1 garlic clove, minced
1 tablespoon salt
½ teaspoon pepper
1 sixteen-ounce can tomatoes, chopped
3 medium potatoes, peeled and cubed
2 onions, chopped
1 package frozen lima beans
1 package frozen corn

In a large kettle with 2 quarts of boiling water, place chicken, ham, hot sauce, garlic, salt, and pepper. Cover and simmer for 45 minutes to 1 hour until chicken is tender. Remove chicken. Debone chicken, shred meat, and set aside. Add tomatoes with their-juice and bring to a boil. Add potatoes, onions, and lima beans. Cover and simmer another 30 minutes or until potatoes are tender. Add chicken and corn. Simmer another 10 minutes.

Serves 8

LIKE THE COLONEL'S CHICKEN

E (*milkless, eggless, glutenless, cornless*)

    1 frying chicken (about 2½
        pounds), cut up, skin removed
    1 cup soy flour
    1 teaspoon paprika
    ¼ cup milkless margarine
        Salt and pepper

Melt margarine in a baking pan. Mix flour, paprika, salt, and pepper in a paper bag. Shake chicken pieces separately in bag until well coated, then place in pan. Bake 1 hour at 400°. Turn chicken over after 30 minutes.

Serves 4–6

CHICKEN CACCIATORE

E (*milkless, eggless, glutenless, cornless*)

    ¼ cup olive or sesame seed oil
    1 frying chicken (2½–3 pounds),
        cut into serving pieces
    ½ cup chopped shallots
    ½ cup sliced mushrooms
    1 garlic clove, minced
    1 cup Chicken Stock* (heat to
        boiling)

    1 sixteen-ounce can tomatoes
    1 six-ounce can tomato paste
    1 teaspoon salt
    ¼ teaspoon white pepper
    ½ teaspoon thyme
    2 bay leaves
        Dash cayenne pepper

Heat oil in a skillet or large frying pan. Add chicken and brown until golden. Add shallots, mushrooms, and garlic, and sauté slightly. Drain off any oil. Add chicken stock, tomatoes, tomato paste, salt, pepper, thyme, bay leaves, and cayenne (not too much). Cover pan and let simmer for 1 hour or until chicken is done. Remove cover for 15–30 minutes until sauce thickens. Serve over rice.

Serves 4

CREAMED ARTICHOKES AND CHICKEN

E (*milkless, eggless, glutenless, cornless*)

4 tablespoons milkless margarine
1 frying chicken (2½ pounds), cut into pieces
2 tablespoons rice flour or potato flour
½ cup chopped shallots
½ cup sliced fresh mushrooms
2 cups Chicken Stock*

1 can artichoke hearts, drained and chopped
1 teaspoon salt
1 cup non-dairy creamer (cornless)
¼ teaspoon lemon pepper

Melt margarine in a large skillet. Coat chicken with flour and fry in skillet until lightly browned. Remove chicken and set aside. Add shallots and mushrooms and sauté until tender. Return chicken to skillet, and add chicken stock, artichoke hearts, salt, and pepper. Simmer covered for 1 hour. Reduce heat and add non-dairy creamer (you may need a little flour to thicken sauce up). Cook until heated thoroughly.

Serves 4

ORANGE CURAÇAO CHICKEN

T (*testing for citrus—milkless, eggless, glutenless*)

1 frying chicken (2½ pounds) cut into serving pieces
¼ cup arrowroot flour
2 tablespoons oil
½ cup sliced fresh mushrooms
1 six-ounce can concentrated orange juice, thawed

4 teaspoons brown sugar
1 tablespoon vinegar
2 tablespoons catsup
2 tablespoons curaçao liqueur
1 tablespoon arrowroot flour mixed with 2 teaspoons water

Coat chicken with flour, then brown in a skillet with oil. Remove chicken and put to one side. Sauté mushrooms in remaining oil. Place chicken and mushrooms in a greased casserole dish. In a small bowl, mix together orange juice, brown sugar, vinegar, catsup, and curaçao. Pour this over chicken and mushrooms, and bake at 350° for 1 to 1½ hours or until chicken is tender. Remove chicken to a warm platter. Thicken sauce with arrowroot and water mixture. Serve over cooked rice. Top with fresh orange slices and parsley sprigs.

NOTE: If preferred, this dish can be made without a liqueur.

Serves 4

CHICKEN PROVENÇAL

E (*milkless, eggless, glutenless, cornless*)

 1 garlic clove, minced
 2 fresh tomatoes, cut into wedges
 ¼ cup Chicken Stock*
 ½ teaspoon thyme
 ½ teaspoon oregano
 ¼ teaspoon rosemary
 1 teaspoon sweet basil
 1 frying chicken (2½ pounds), cut
   into serving pieces
 ¼ cup soy flour
 ½ teaspoon salt
 ⅛ teaspoon pepper
 ¼ cup sunflower oil
 1 eight-ounce can chopped black
   olives

In a saucepan combine garlic, tomatoes, stock, and spices. Simmer for 1 hour until mixture thickens. In a small paper sack, place soy flour, salt, and pepper. Shake chicken pieces in flour mixture, then brown in skillet with oil. Grease a 1-quart casserole or a 9 × 13-inch baking pan. Arrange chicken in bottom of pan and pour sauce over chicken. Sprinkle olives on top and bake at 350° for 1 hour.

Serves 4

CHICKEN AND DUMPLINGS

(*milkless, cornless*)

1 chicken, 2½–3½ pounds
2 cups Chicken Stock*
½ cup chopped onion
½ cup chopped celery
4 medium carrots, sliced
1 teaspoon salt
½ teaspoon pepper

Dumplings:
1 cup flour
1½ tablespoons baking powder
1 teaspoon salt
¼ teaspoon sage
1 tablespoon minced parsley
1 egg
⅓ cup soy milk
2 teaspoons sesame seed oil

In a large casserole or baking dish, combine the chicken, vegetables, stock, and seasoning and bake at 400° for 1 hour.

To make the dumplings, combine egg, milk, oil, parsley, and sage in a small mixing bowl. Add flour, baking powder, and salt. Stir and blend until dry ingredients are moistened. Place in small drops over top of stew in the casserole dish. Bake an additional 20–30 minutes at same oven setting.

Serves 6

CHICKEN WITH PEACHES

E (*milkless, eggless, glutenless, cornless*)

1 chicken, 1–2½ pounds, cut into
  pieces
4 tablespoons milkless margarine
  Salt and pepper to taste
½ cup chopped onion

3 tablespoons brown sugar
1 cup Chicken Stock*
4 peaches (firm, fresh, or canned
  packed in own juices)

Prepare chicken. In a large skillet, melt margarine. Add chicken and brown lightly. Season with salt and pepper. Remove from heat, and set aside. Add onions and sauté until tender. Add brown sugar and chicken stock, and bring to a boil. Place chicken in a 1½-quart casserole dish. Peel peaches, remove pits, cut them into large wedges, and arrange over chicken. Pour sauce over all. Cover and bake at 350° for 30 minutes.

Serves 4

CHINESE CHICKEN BREASTS

E (*milkless, eggless, glutenless, cornless*)

1½ to 2 pounds chicken breasts, boned and cooked
2 tablespoons sesame seed oil
2 tablespoons tapioca flour
¼ cup water
1 tablespoon tamari (traditional/ wheat-free)
1 cup chopped celery
½ cup chopped onion
¼ cup sliced shallots

½ cup chopped green pepper
1 cup Chinese peas
½ cup sliced mushrooms
1 can water chestnuts
2 cups bean sprouts
½ cup blanched almonds
¼ teaspoon salt
⅛ teaspoon pepper

Slice cooked chicken into small pieces. Brown slightly in a large skillet with oil. Add celery and onions, and sauté until tender. Add green pepper, peas, mushrooms, water chestnuts, bean sprouts, almonds, salt, and pepper. Cook until vegetables are chewy but not tender.

In a small mixing bowl, mix tapioca flour, water, and tamari. Cook over medium heat until thoroughly heated; then pour over vegetables and chicken, mixing well. Serve with steamed rice.

Serves 4

CHICKEN WITH RAISIN SAUCE

E (*milkless, eggless, glutenless, cornless*)

4 chicken breasts, deboned and skinned
1 teaspoon arrowroot flour
3 tablespoons brown sugar
½ teaspoon oregano
1 clove garlic

2 tablespoons safflower oil
3 tablespoons tamari (traditional/ wheat-free)
½ cup Chicken Stock*
½ cup raisins

Place chicken breasts in a greased skillet. Mix together remaining ingredients and pour over chicken breasts. Bring sauce to a boil, then reduce heat to simmer for 45 minutes or until chicken is tender. Serve over rice.

Serves 4

CHICKEN DIVAN

T (*testing for gluten—milkless, eggless, cornless*)

4 breasts of chicken, skinned,
  boned, cooked, and sliced
½ pound fresh broccoli
2 teaspoons milkless margarine
½ cup chopped onion
2 tablespoons arrowroot
2 cups Cream of Chicken soup*
½ teaspoon salt
½ teaspoon curry
½ cup soft wheat bread crumbs
2 tablespoons milkless margarine,
  melted

Prepare chicken breasts and set aside. In a saucepan, cook broccoli in one cup of water until just tender. In a separate saucepan, melt margarine. Add onions and sauté until tender. Add arrowroot, salt, and then mushroom soup. Cook until thickened. Add curry powder.

Place broccoli in greased 9 × 13-inch baking pan. Layer sliced cooked chicken on top. Pour heated sauce over broccoli and chicken. Sprinkle with bread crumbs and pour melted margarine over all. Bake covered in a preheated 375° oven for 30–35 minutes.

Serves 4–6

SPINACH CHICKEN BREASTS

E (*milkless, eggless, glutenless, cornless*)

3 tablespoons safflower oil
6 chicken breasts, boned
¼ cup chopped shallots
1½ cups tapioca flour mixed with
  ¼ cup potato flour
1 pound fresh spinach, chopped
½ tablespoon chopped fresh dill,
  or ½ teaspoon dried dill

½ tablespoon chopped fresh
  fennel, or ½ teaspoon dried
  fennel
⅛ teaspoon salt
⅛ teaspoon black pepper
⅛ teaspoon nutmeg
2 to 3 ounces crumbled Feta cheese
  (imported/goat)
1 cup hot Chicken Stock*

Skin chicken breasts and pound until thin. Dip each breast in flour mixture, and brown in a skillet with hot oil. Remove chicken and set aside on a warm platter. Add shallots and sauté until tender. Wash and clean spinach. Add chopped spinach, dill, fennel, salt, pepper, and nutmeg to skillet and stir together. Place chicken breasts in an 8 × 8-inch casserole dish, and spoon spinach mixture over them. Place Feta cheese on top of spinach mixture, and pour hot stock over all. Place in a 375° oven and bake until Feta is melted, about 40 minutes.

Serves 4

CHICKEN STEW

E (milkless, eggless, glutenless, cornless)

2 tablespoons milkless margarine
1 stewing chicken, cut up
½ cup chopped onions
1 sixteen-ounce can tomatoes, chopped (save liquid)
½ cup Chicken Stock*

1 teaspoon salt
3 peppercorns
1 sixteen-ounce can garbanzo beans
½ cup chopped almonds
½ cup boiling water (optional)

In a large saucepan or skillet, melt margarine, add chicken, and brown until golden. Add onion and sauté until tender. Add tomatoes (drained with liquid saved), chicken stock, salt, peppercorns, and enough liquid from the canned tomatoes to cover. Simmer chicken for 1 hour. Mix garbanzo beans with remaining tomato liquid or a little boiling water and add to chicken. Mix well. Stir in almonds and cook for 10 minutes more. Serve hot in bowls.

Serves 8

CHICKEN ROLLS

T (testing for pork—eggless, glutenless, cornless)

3 whole chicken breasts, skinned and boned
6 small slices of ham
6 small slices Swiss cheese
¼ cup soy flour
3 tablespoons grated Romano cheese (imported/sheep)
1 teaspoon salt

¼ teaspoon pepper
½ teaspoon powdered sage
¼ teaspoon thyme
⅓ cup sesame seed oil
1 cup Chicken Stock*
2 envelopes of dry Lipton cream of chicken soup (has potato base)

Cut each boned chicken breast in half, and pound until thin between 2 sheets of waxed paper or foil. Cut each chicken breast in half lengthwise. Place a slice of cheese and a slice of ham on each piece of chicken. Roll each and secure with a toothpick. Dip chicken rolls into a mixture of soy flour, cheese, salt, pepper, sage, and thyme. Refrigerate for 30 minutes to 1 hour. In a large skillet, heat oil and brown chicken on all sides. Place browned chicken in a slow-cooking pot. Add soup mixed with chicken stock. Cover and cook over low heat for 5–6 hours. Turn heat to high, and thicken sauce with leftover flour and cheese mixture. Cook over high heat for 15 minutes. Serve with rice.

NOTE: Lipton soup contains MSG (monosodium glutamate).

Serves 6

CHICKEN A LA KING

T (*testing for gluten—milkless, eggless, cornless*)

2 cups chicken, cooked and cubed
3 tablespoons milkless margarine
½ cup unsifted all-purpose flour
1½ cups milk substitute (see Appendix A)
½ cup Chicken Stock*

¼ cup sliced shallots
½ cup sliced fresh mushrooms
¼ cup chopped green pepper
1 four-ounce jar chopped pimento
1 teaspoon salt
¼ teaspoon pepper

Melt margarine in a skillet. Sauté shallots until tender. Add flour and stir until well blended. Slowly add milk substitute and stock. Add chicken, mushrooms, green pepper, pimento, salt, and pepper. Simmer over medium heat for 15 minutes. Serve over milkless, eggless toast or rice.

Serves 4–6

ROAST TURKEY

E (*milkless, eggless, glutenless, cornless—if unstuffed or stuffed with Rice Stuffing*)

Use Tom Turkey only. Remove stuffings from body cavity and neck cavity; rinse inside and out with cold water; dry. Salt inside of both cavities, and stuff with prepared stuffing just before roasting. Close body cavity with skewers and lace with string. Place on a rack in a shallow open pan breast-side up. Brush skin of bird with milkless margarine. Roast according to weight of bird. Remove skin before serving.

HOT TURKEY SANDWICHES

E (*milkless, eggless, glutenless, cornless*)

1 pound sliced turkey   Turkey Gravy*
  Rice bread,* sliced

Heat turkey slices. Mix turkey gravy, and pour over turkey slices and bread. Serve hot.

Serves 4

TURKEY GRAVY

E (*milkless, eggless, glutenless, cornless*)

½ cup milkless margarine (or
  turkey drippings)
4 tablespoons arrowroot flour (or
  2 tablespoons potato flour and
  1 tablespoon tapioca flour)
½ cup Chicken Stock*
½ teaspoon salt
¼ teaspoon pepper
2 cups milk substitute (see
  Appendix A)
1 teaspoon poultry seasoning

Melt margarine in a saucepan. Add flour slowly and cook until well blended. Slowly add stock and milk, stirring well. Season. Cook, stirring slowly, until thick.

Makes 2 cups

TURKEY GOULASH

T (*testing for milk—eggless, glutenless, cornless*)

3 cups cooked, chopped turkey
1 cup chopped onion
1 clove garlic, pressed
1¾ cups Chicken Stock*
1 cup tomato sauce

1 tablespoon paprika
1 teaspoon salt
⅛ teaspoon pepper
1 cup sour cream
2 tablespoons margarine

Melt margarine in a large skillet, and sauté onion and garlic. Add turkey, stock, tomato sauce, and seasonings. Simmer for 10 minutes. Remove from heat and stir in sour cream. Serve over rice.

Serves 6

TURKEY TETRAZZINI

T (*testing for citrus—milkless, eggless, cornless*)

¼ cup milkless margarine
1 pound sliced mushrooms
½ cup chopped onions
1 tablespoon lemon juice
1 teaspoon salt
1 teaspoon paprika

¼ cup arrowroot flour
1¾ cups Chicken Stock*
½ cup soy milk
3 cups cubed turkey
1 seven-ounce package spaghetti, cooked

Melt margarine in a skillet. Sauté mushrooms and onions. Stir in flour, then slowly add soy milk, stock, and seasonings. Simmer for 15 minutes, then add turkey. Place cooked spaghetti in a greased 1½-quart casserole. Pour turkey mixture over spaghetti, and bake for 20 minutes at 350°.

Serves 4

VEGETARIAN DISHES

TOFU-STUFFED ARTICHOKES

(milkless, glutenless, cornless)

10 large globe artichokes
¼ teaspoon salt
½ teaspoon minced garlic
2 tablespoons milkless margarine
½ cup chopped onion
1 pound tofu, cubed
⅛ teaspoon pepper
2 tablespoons freshly chopped
    parsley

¼ cup rice bread* crumbs
2 eggs (or substitute, see
    Appendix A)
1½ cups Béchamel Sauce*
2 tablespoons freshly grated
    Romano cheese (imported/
    sheep)

Prepare artichokes. Remove outer leaves, cut off tops, and remove chokes. Place artichokes in 2 inches of water in a large 8-quart saucepan or dutch oven. Sprinkle salt and garlic over artichokes and cook covered until tender.

In a large skillet, melt margarine, and sauté onions until tender. Beat 1 egg and add to the mixture. Blend in bread crumbs, tofu, pepper, and parsley and mix. Add Béchamel sauce, second egg, and cheese. Mix well. Spoon some of the mixture into each artichoke. Place in a 9 × 13-inch baking dish. Bake at 350° for 40 minutes.

Serves 10

BEAN STEW

E (*milkless, eggless, glutenless, cornless*)

4 tablespoons milkless margarine
1 cup chopped onions
1 garlic clove, minced
1 pound green beans
1 cup water

2 fresh tomatoes, skinned and
chopped, or 1 small can tomatoes
1 teaspoon salt
¼ teaspoon pepper
1 tablespoon tamari (traditional/
wheat-free)

Melt margarine in a saucepan. Sauté onion and garlic until tender. Cut beans in half lengthwise, and add to onion and garlic. Steam for about 30 minutes, stirring occasionally. Add tomatoes and water just to cover beans. Add salt and pepper and cook until tender. Add tamari the last 15 minutes.

Serves 4

VEGETARIAN CABBAGE ROLLS

E (*milkless, eggless, glutenless, cornless*)

1 head of white cabbage
1 fifteen-ounce can garbanzo
beans
1 small can sliced olives
1 cup rice, washed
1 bunch parsley, chopped
½ cup pine nuts
½ cup chopped onion
¼ cup chopped shallots
1¼ teaspoon salt

⅛ teaspoon pepper
Dash cayenne pepper (not much)
½ teaspoon allspice
½ teaspoon anise seed
¼ teaspoon ground cinnamon
¼ teaspoon nutmeg
1 sixteen-ounce can whole
tomatoes, chopped
½ cup water
1 fifteen-ounce can tomato sauce

Cut out center core of cabbage. Boil cabbage head in a large kettle just long enough to soften and separate leaves. Tear off leaves and set aside to drain. In a large mixing bowl, combine garbanzo beans, olives, rice, parsley, pine nuts, onion, shallots and seasonings. Stuff each cabbage leaf with a little of the garbanzo bean mixture. Fold in ends of leaves, then roll. Arrange side-by-side in a covered kettle. Pour tomatoes and water over top of cabbage leaves, and steam over low heat until done.

Serves 8

CARROT FRITTERS

(milkless, glutenless, cornless)

2 tablespoons milkless margarine
2 medium shallots, thinly sliced
1 garlic clove, minced
¼ cup soy flour
2 tablespoons chopped parsley

½ teaspoon salt
⅛ teaspoon pepper
1 tablespoon lemon juice
2 eggs, beaten
3 cups shredded carrots

Melt margarine in a large skillet, and sauté shallots and garlic. In a medium-size bowl, combine flour, parsley, salt, pepper, and lemon juice. Add shallots and garlic, then stir in eggs and carrots. Drop mixture by tablespoon onto a lightly greased skillet. Cook for about 5 minutes on each side or until brown.

Makes 12–15

CHILES RELLENOS CASSEROLE

(glutenless, cornless)

2 four-ounce cans whole green
chiles, washed and dried
1½ cups shredded Monterey Jack
cheese

2 eggs, beaten
1 tablespoon tapioca flour
1 tablespoon potato flour

Place whole green chiles into a greased 8 × 2-inch casserole dish. Sprinkle cheese on top and pour in beaten eggs mixed with tapioca flour and potato flour. Bake at 350° for 30–35 minutes.

Serves 6

CHINESE CABBAGE STEW

E *(milkless, eggless, glutenless, cornless)*

2 tablespoons sesame oil
2 cups thinly sliced onions
½ cup sliced carrots
½ cup chopped celery
3 medium potatoes, diced

2 cups sliced Chinese cabbage
3 cups water
2 tablespoons tamari (traditional/
wheat-free)
2 tablespoons minced parsley

Heat oil in a large kettle. Add onion, carrots, celery, and Chinese cabbage, and sauté until tender. Add water and bring to a boil. Reduce heat, cover and simmer for 20 minutes. Stir in tamari and parsley. Cool overnight. Reheat in 8 hours and serve.

Serves 4

LIMA BEAN CASSEROLE

T (*testing for milk—eggless, glutenless, cornless*)

2 tablespoons margarine
1 garlic clove, minced
½ cup chopped shallots
½ cup peeled and grated carrots
¼ cup chopped fresh parsley
1 ten-ounce package frozen lima beans

1 cup tomato juice
½ cup water
½ cup rice bread* crumbs
½ cup Parmesan cheese
½ teaspoon salt

In a 10-inch skillet, melt margarine. Add garlic, shallots, and carrots, and sauté until tender. Add parsley and lima beans. Mix tomato juice with water. Pour into skillet until liquid is just covering beans. Transfer to a 1½-quart casserole, and bake covered at 350° for 45 minutes. Top with bread crumbs and Parmesan cheese. Bake for 10 minutes more uncovered, or until topping is just golden brown.

Serves 4

PINTO CHILI

E (*milkless, eggless, glutenless, cornless*)

2 cups raw pinto beans
3½ cups canned tomatoes
¾ cup tomato paste

1 tablespoon chili powder
1 teaspoon chopped garlic
1 tablespoon salt

Cook pinto beans in 6 cups of boiling water for 2 minutes. Let sit 1 hour. Cook until tender (4 hours on stove, 8 hours in a crock pot). Add tomatoes, tomato paste, and seasonings. Cook slowly about 1 hour before serving.

Serves 12

SPINACH WITH RICE

E (*milkless, eggless, glutenless, cornless*)

1 pound spinach	¼ cup rice
2 medium onions, chopped	¼ cup olive oil
1 tablespoon each chopped	Salt and pepper to taste
parsley and dill	

Sauté onions in heated oil until golden. Drain excess oil. Add spinach, which has been thoroughly washed and drained. Add a little water and bring to a boil. Sprinkle on parsley and dill and add washed rice. Stir, season to taste, cover, and allow to simmer for 15 minutes or until tender.

Serves 4

SPINACH PIE

T (*testing for eggs—milkless, glutenless, cornless*)

1 nine-inch Basic Rice Pie Crust*
2½ pounds spinach
¼ cup olive oil
1 onion, chopped
1 cup freshly chopped mint
1 pound crumbled Feta cheese
  (imported/goat)
6 eggs, separated (room
  temperature)
Salt and pepper

Clean and wash spinach. Pat dry with paper towel, and chop. In a 10-inch skillet, heat oil, add onion and sauté until tender. Drain oil. In a large mixing bowl, combine sautéd onion, mint, and spinach. Add Feta cheese, salt, and pepper. Add egg yolks and mix thoroughly. Beat egg whites until stiff but not dry. Mix one-quarter into spinach mixture, then gently fold remaining egg whites into mixture. Pour into pie crust and bake at 400° for about 35–40 minutes. Allow to cool.

Serves 4–6

SQUASH PIE

T (*testing for eggs—milkless, glutenless, cornless*)

1 Basic Rice Pie Crust*
2½ pounds chopped squash
 (zucchini, yellow squash, etc.)
1 cup finely chopped onions
1 tablespoon milkless margarine
⅓ cup olive oil

½ cup rice
1 cup boiling water
10 eggs, beaten
½ pound grated cheese (Kassari
 or Kefalotysi) (imported/
 sheep)

Prepare pie crust in a 9-inch pie pan. Set aside. In a large 10-inch skillet, sauté onions in margarine and olive oil until tender. Drain excess oil. Add rice and boiling water to skillet. Cover and cook over low heat until done, about 15 minutes. Do not peek. Steam squash in saucepan with water until just cooked; remove from heat and allow to cool. Combine eggs and cheese with squash mixture, then mix cooked rice into squash mixture. Pour into prepared pie crust. Bake at 350° for 15 minutes, then reduce to 325° for an additional 30 minutes.

Serves 4–6

STUFFED TOMATOES WITH RICE

E (*milkless, eggless, glutenless, cornless*)

10 large tomatoes
1 cup rice
1 onion, chopped
5 cloves garlic, chopped
¼ cup chopped dill
 Salt and pepper to taste
¼ cup parsley, chopped

¼ cup tomato paste
¼ cup water
½ cup olive oil
1 tablespoon sugar
2 cups pulp and juice scooped
 from the tomatoes

Slice off tops and scoop out tomatoes. Discard hard center. Place tomatoes in a baking pan. Mix remaining ingredients together and spoon into tomato cups. Replace tops. Pour in enough boiling water to cover bottom of pan. Cover and bake at 350° for 45 minutes, then uncover and bake until brown and done.

NOTE: Green peppers may be used in place of tomatoes.

Serves 8–10

STUFFED TOMATOES WITH CHEESE

E (*milkless, eggless, glutenless, cornless*)

6 ripe tomatoes
1½ teaspoons salt
1 cup fresh basil leaves, or
   4 tablespoons dried basil
½ cup almonds, chopped
2 tablespoons grated Romano

cheese (imported/sheep)
¼ cup crushed Feta cheese
   (imported/goat)
1 eight-ounce can garbanzo
   beans, drained
Paprika

Cut tops off and scoop out pulp from tomatoes. In a blender or food processor combine basil, almonds, Romano, Feta, and garbanzo beans until smooth and creamy. Spoon into each tomato. Sprinkle with paprika.

Serves 6

BASIC FRITTER RECIPE

(*milkless, cornless*)

3 eggs, separated
2 tablespoons safflower oil

3 tablespoons flour
½ teaspoon water

Beat egg yolks together with oil. Stir in flour and salt. Add just enough water to make a thick creamy batter. Beat egg whites until stiff, but not dry, and fold them in. Stir or dip vegetables in batter and drop into hot oil. Cook until golden brown. Drain on paper towels.

Serves 4

SWISS CHARD PIE

(*milkless, glutenless, cornless*)

½ cup chopped mushrooms
1 small onion, chopped
¼ cup milkless margarine
30 leaves of Swiss chard, torn into
   pieces

2 eggs, slightly beaten
½ cup grated cheese (your choice,
   sheep or goat)
⅓ cup chopped green chiles or
   green bell pepper

Preheat oven to 350°. Sauté onions and mushrooms in margarine until onions are transparent. Add chard and cook 1 minute or until it wilts. Be sure chard is well covered with margarine. Pour into pie pan. Mix eggs with green chiles and pour over chard. Stir around with a fork. Spread cheese on top and bake until firm.

Serves 6–8

BAKED VEGETABLE DINNER

E (*milkless, eggless, glutenless, cornless*)

1 pound potatoes	¼ cup chopped parsley
1 pound okra, or string beans	Salt and pepper to taste
1 pound squash	1 cup olive oil
1 pound tomatoes	1 sprig of dill
1 pound onions	

Peel and prepare vegetables; slice potatoes, onions, squash, and okra. Arrange vegetables in layers, sprinkling a little dill, parsley, salt, pepper, and olive oil between each layer. Add a little water and bake in a moderate oven for 1 hour.

Serves 4–6

VEGETARIAN PIZZA

T (*testing for milk—eggless, glutenless, cornless*)

Pizza dough:
Look for a package of commercial gluten-free brown rice baking mix that has a recipe for pizza on the back.

Sauce:
In a saucepan, combine 2 cups tomato sauce, 1 teaspoon oregano, 1 teaspoon Italian seasoning, ¼ cup water, 1 teaspoon thyme, ½ teaspoon garlic salt, and salt and pepper. Heat until boiling. Reduce heat and allow to thicken.

Topping:

2 green peppers, sliced	½ onion, sliced
1 four-ounce can black olives, sliced	1⅔ cups shredded Mozzarella cheese
½ pound fresh mushrooms, sliced	½ cup grated Parmesan cheese

Prepare pizza dough as instructed on box of brown rice baking mix. Spread out on a pizza pan. Pour sauce on top. Top with Mozzarella cheese, mushrooms, green peppers, and olives. Finish with grated Parmesan cheese. Bake at 425° for 40 minutes.

Serves 4–6

VEGETARIAN STEW

E (*milkless, eggless, glutenless, cornless*)

2 tablespoons milkless margarine
1 red onion, chopped
1 teaspoon thyme
Bouquet Garni*
4 cups tomato juice
1 turnip, peeled and chopped
1 cup sliced celery
1 pound red potatoes, peeled and cut in chunks
6 carrots, peeled, washed, cut in half and then julienned
1 fifteen-ounce can garbanzo beans
1 cup rice bread* crumbs
2 tablespoons chopped parsley
½ cup grated Kassari cheese (imported/sheep)

In a large casserole dish, melt margarine; add onion and thyme, and sauté. Add bouquet garni, tomato juice, turnip, celery, potatoes, and carrots. Bring to a boil. Cover and simmer 30 minutes, or until potatoes and carrots are just tender. Uncover and add garbanzo beans. Cook and reduce liquid. Top with bread crumbs and cheese, and sprinkle with parsley.

Serves 4–6

VEGETABLE TEMPURA

E (*milkless, eggless, glutenless, cornless*)

Allowed vegetables: asparagus spears, green onions, cauliflower, sweet potatoes, mushrooms, green peppers, zucchini and squash.

Cooking Oil: Safflower oil

Tempura:
¾ cup flour (arrowroot, soy, rice)
½ cup cold water, include some ice cubes
1 egg substitute (see Appendix A)

2 tablespoons safflower oil
½ teaspoon salt

Condiment Mixture:
2 tablespoons tamari (traditional/ wheat-free)
¼ cup prepared mustard

Combine flour, oil, egg substitute, and salt. Mix in cold water (along with some ice cubes). Dip cut vegetables into batter and then fry in hot oil until light brown. Drain on paper towel. Serve with condiment mixture.

Serves 4

VEGEBURGER

E (*milkless, eggless, glutenless, cornless*)

2 cups cooked and mashed pinto
  or navy beans
1 cup cooked brown or white rice
½ cup shredded carrots
¼ cup chopped onions
1 egg substitute (see Appendix A)
1 teaspoon sea salt

¼ teaspoon ground pepper
2 tablespoons parsley flakes
½ teaspoon garlic salt
½ teaspoon Italian seasoning (see
  Ingredient Glossary under
  Herbs and Spices) or ½ teaspoon
  tamari

Mix together above ingredients, and form into patties. Barbecue or pan fry. Serve over rice bread or separately.

Variation: Avocado Burger: Mash 2 peeled and pitted avocados and add ½ cup chopped almonds instead of first two ingredients listed.

NOTE: Navy or pinto beans need to cook slowly for 8 hours in a crock pot or 4 hours, approximately, on a regular stove.

Makes 4–6 patties

ZUCCHINI BOATS

E (*milkless, eggless, glutenless, cornless*)

4 medium zucchini
¼ cup milkless margarine
¼ cup chopped green onions
½ pound fresh mushrooms,
  chopped
1 cup chopped almonds
½ cup water chestnuts
1 cup rice bread* crumbs

2 tablespoons chopped parsley
1 tablespoon paprika
1 tablespoon tamari (traditional/
  wheat-free)

Cut zucchini in half lengthwise. Boil until tender; drain and cool. Scoop out zucchini and mash, reserving the shells. Melt margarine in a skillet, and sauté onions and mushrooms until tender. In a mixing bowl, mix mashed zucchini with mushrooms and onion. Add almonds, chestnuts, bread crumbs, parsley, and tamari. Place zucchini boats in a low pan, and fill each boat with some zucchini mixture. Bake 20 minutes at 350°.

Serves 6

CHEESE AND EGG DISHES

CHEESE SAUCE

E (*milkless, eggless, glutenless, cornless*)

¼ cup freshly grated Romano
   cheese (imported/sheep)
1 cup Eggless Mayonnaise I*
   (or see Appendix A)
1 tablespoon soy baby formula
   (cornless)
1 tablespoon finely chopped fresh
   mushrooms

1 tablespoon capers
1 teaspoon finely chopped onion
½ teaspoon salt
½ teaspoon dill weed
¼ teaspoon paprika
¼ teaspoon pepper

Mix all ingredients together with a whisk. Cover and chill for 2 hours.

Makes 1½ cups

FRESH BASIL PESTO

E (*milkless, eggless, glutenless, cornless*)

1½ cups fresh basil leaves, packed
2 large garlic cloves, peeled
3 tablespoons freshly grated
   Romano cheese (imported/
   sheep)
3 tablespoons olive oil

Put basil and garlic into a mortar and, using a grinding motion, crush ingredients with a pestle into a fine paste. Blend in cheese, continuing to grind until mixture is well blended. Add oil bit by bit, mixing with the pestle until you have a smooth paste.

With a blender or food processor, combine basil and garlic and blend to a fine paste. Add cheese and process or blend until smooth. Add oil bit by bit, turning on machine after each addition and mixing until smooth and creamy.

Transfer pesto to a jar. Cover with a thin layer of olive oil. Seal jar and store in refrigerator.

Makes 1 cup

KASSARI CHEESE PUFFS

(*milkless, glutenless, cornless*)

1 pound Kassari cheese
   (imported/sheep)
2 egg whites
⅛ teaspoon white pepper

⅛ teaspoon oregano
1 tablespoon minced parsley
Safflower oil

Grate cheese. Beat egg whites into peaks that are stiff but not dry. Mix cheese with pepper, oregano, and parsley. Mix one-quarter of egg whites into cheese mixture, then gently fold in remaining egg whites. Roll into 1-inch balls and fry quickly in hot oil until golden brown.

Serves 8

KASSARI FRITTERS

(*milkless, glutenless, cornless*)

2 eggs
1 cup grated Kassari (imported/
   sheep)

1 teaspoon tamari (traditional/
   wheat-free)
2 tablespoons milkless margarine

Beat eggs well, then add grated cheese and tamari. In a 10-inch skillet, melt the margarine. Spoon mixture into skillet to form 4 1-inch circles. Cook as pancakes, until each side is lightly brown.

Serves 8

KASSARI SPREAD

E (*milkless, eggless, glutenless, cornless*)

½ cup grated Kassari cheese
(imported/sheep)
½ cup tofu, mashed
2 tablespoons chopped and seeded
green chiles

2 tablespoons chopped pimento
½ cup Eggless Mayonnaise I*
(or see Appendix A)

In a medium-size mixing bowl, combine ingredients. Mix with a whisk until creamy. Use paste as a spread on toasted rice bread or rice crackers.

Makes 1 cup

TOFU CROQUETTES

(*milkless, glutenless, cornless*)

2 cups tofu, mashed
1 tablespoon safflower oil
½ teaspoon salt
2 tablespoons finely chopped
onion
2 cups cooked rice

4 tablespoons freshly chopped
parsley
1 tablespoon tamari (traditional/
wheat-free)
1 egg, beaten
rice cereal. crushed

Mix all ingredients together thoroughly except the cereal. Roll mixture into small balls. Dip croquettes in beaten egg, and then in crushed cereal. Place croquettes on a greased 9 × 13-inch pan. Bake at 400° for 30 minutes.

Makes 1½ dozen

ROQUEFORT CHEESE MOLD

T (*testing for eggs—milkless, glutenless, cornless*)

4 ounces Roquefort cheese,
crumbled (imported/sheep)
¼ cup white wine vinegar
¼ cup chopped fresh parsley
2 tablespoons chopped onion
⅛ teaspoon white pepper
2 tablespoons poppy seeds

1 cup peeled and very finely
chopped cucumber
½ cup soy milk
4 ounces tofu
3 egg whites, stiffly beaten
1 envelope unflavored gelatin
¼ cup cold water

Force Roquefort through a fine sieve or process in a blender or food processor without liquifying. Combine with vinegar, parsley, onion, white pepper, and poppy seeds. Add chopped cucumber, soy milk, and tofu and mix well. In a separate bowl, beat egg whites until stiff but not dry. Fold egg whites into Roquefort mixture. Soften gelatin in cold water in cup. Place cup in a pan of hot water and dissolve gelatin, then stir into cheese mixture. Pour into an oiled 2-quart mold and chill at least 2 hours. Unmold onto a platter and garnish.

Serves 8

MUSHROOM QUICHE

(milkless, glutenless, cornless)

1 nine-inch pastry shell (Basic Rice* or Kassari Cheese*)
3 tablespoons milkless margarine
½ cup sliced shallots
½ cup sliced mushrooms
1 tablespoon arrowroot flour
3 eggs, slightly beaten (no substitutes)

8 ounces tofu
½ teaspoon salt
⅛ teaspoon pepper
Dash of nutmeg
⅓ cup freshly grated Romano cheese (imported/sheep)

Prepare pastry shell according to instructions and bake in a 450° oven for 7 minutes. In a large skillet, melt margarine and sauté shallots and mushrooms. Blend in flour, eggs, tofu, salt, pepper, and nutmeg. Pour mixture into the pastry shell. Sprinkle with Romano cheese and bake in a 350° oven for 30–35 minutes.

Serves 8

TOFU QUICHE

(milkless, glutenless, cornless)

2 tablespoons milkless margarine
½ cup chopped onion
¼ cup chopped green pepper
½ cup sliced mushrooms
4 large eggs, beaten
1 cup milk substitute (see Appendix A)

½ cup tofu, mashed
⅔ cup grated Romano cheese (imported/sheep)
⅛ teaspoon nutmeg
Salt and pepper
1 baked 8- or 9-inch pastry shell (Basic Rice* or Kassari Cheese*)

In a large skillet, melt margarine, and sauté onions and green pepper until just tender. In a large mixing bowl, mix together mushrooms, eggs, soy milk, tofu, cheese, salt, pepper, and nutmeg. Add onions and green peppers. Mix well. Pour into pastry shell, and bake at 400°–425° for 20–25 minutes.

Serves 8

ZUCCHINI FRITTER

(milkless, glutenless, cornless)

2 zucchini, peeled and cubed
¼ cup potato starch
3 tablespoons milkless margarine
5 eggs, slightly beaten

1 tablespoon grated Romano cheese (imported/sheep)
½ teaspoon salt
¼ teaspoon pepper
⅛ teaspoon oregano

Prepare zucchini. In a large skillet, melt margarine. Dip zucchini pieces in flour, then sauté until tender. In a large mixing bowl, mix together well the cooked zucchini, eggs, grated cheese, salt, pepper, and oregano. Pour zucchini mixture into skillet, and cook until lightly brown on each side.

Serves 6

RICE DISHES

TIPS ON COOKING RICE

1. Rice, except in a few cases, should not be stirred while cooking.
2. Cook rice on low heat after water has boiled. Do not look at it while cooking.
3. Once rice is cooked, remove it from the heat source and let steam.

BOILED RICE:

Method I
1 cup rice
2 cups boiling water
2 tablespoons milkless margarine
Salt

Bring water, margarine, and salt to a boil. Add rice, stir once, lower heat, and cook covered for 20 minutes. No stirring. Remove from heat and let steam 5 minutes.

Method II (oven-boiled rice)
1 cup rice   1 tablespoon salt
2 cups boiling water

Heat oven to 350°. Mix above ingredients together and pour into 1–2-quart casserole dish. Cover and bake 25–30 minutes until rice is tender. Do not peek!

Serves 4

RISOTTO

E (*milkless, eggless, glutenless, cornless*)

2 tablespoons milkless margarine
2 tablespoons olive oil
1 cup raw rice

¼ cup chopped onion
1 clove garlic, minced
3 cups Chicken or Beef Stock*

Melt margarine in a 10-inch skillet. Add oil and uncooked rice and stir well to coat grains. Let rice brown slightly. Add onion and garlic, and sauté until tender. Add stock; cover and lower heat to a simmer. Simmer 20–30 minutes until rice is tender.

Serves 4

WHITE RICE (Japanese style)

E (*milkless, eggless, glutenless, cornless*)

2 cups uncooked white rice
2½ cups water

1 teaspoon tamari (traditional/ wheat-free)

Wash rice in a sieve or colander until water is clear. Place rinsed rice in a saucepan, add water, and let stand for 20 minutes. Cover pan tightly and place on high heat. Cook until water boils and foams, about 5 minutes. Reduce heat and cook 5–10 minutes more until all water is absorbed. Increase heat to high and cook for 30 seconds. Remove pan from heat and let stand 5 minutes.

Serves 4

CHINESE FRIED RICE

(*milkless, glutenless, cornless*)

5 tablespoons milkless margarine
½ cup chopped shallots
½ cup slivered almonds
½ cup sliced celery
½ cup chopped green pepper
½ cup sliced mushrooms (optional if you suspect yeast allergy)

1 eight-ounce can water chestnuts, drained and sliced
2 eggs, slightly beaten
3 cups cooked rice
2 tablespoons tamari (traditional/ wheat-free)

In a large skillet, melt 2 tablespoons margarine, and sauté shallots, almonds, celery, green peppers, and mushrooms. Transfer mixture from skillet into a mixing bowl, and add water chestnuts. Heat 2 additional tablespoons of margarine in skillet, add eggs and stir lightly until set. Remove eggs from skillet and slice into strips. Add remaining tablespoon of margarine and rice and stir-fry until well heated. Add vegetable mixture and sliced eggs to rice and stir in tamari. Stir-fry 1–2 minutes until heated throughly.

Serves 4

CONFETTI RICE

E (*milkless, eggless, glutenless, cornless*)

¼ cup milkless margarine	¼ cup chopped green pepper
2 cups cooked rice	1 teaspoon paprika
½ cup grated carrots	2 tablespoons chopped onion
¼ cup chopped pimentos	¼ cup water

Melt margarine in a skillet, and sauté green peppers, onions, carrots, and pimento until tender. Add water, and simmer 5 minutes. Toss with cooked rice and serve.

Serves 4

MAI FUN FOR SALAD

(*Rice Sticks/Rice Vermicelli*)
E (*milkless, eggless, glutenless, cornless*)

3 handfuls of rice sticks
  Safflower oil (enough to be 3 inches
  deep in a saucepan)

Heat a large frying pan or wok to 350–375°. Break rice sticks into 3-inch lengths. Dip a portion of the sticks into hot oil. They will puff up in a few seconds. Turn noodles over to cook evenly. As soon as noodles stop crackling, remove them to paper towels to drain. Use immediately or store in an air-tight container for a few weeks.

CURRIED RICE

E (*milkless, eggless, glutenless, cornless*)

2 tablespoons milkless margarine
¼ cup chopped onion
½ teaspoon curry powder
¼ teaspoon pepper

½ teaspoon salt
3 cups cooked rice
½ cup chopped blanched almonds

In a 10-inch skillet, melt margarine, and sauté onion until tender. Add curry, pepper, salt, and cooked rice and stir well. Cook until thoroughly heated. Sprinkle almonds over the rice mixture. Serve hot.

Serves 4

FRIED RICE ALMONDINE

E (*milkless, eggless, glutenless, cornless*)

1 cup brown rice
½ cup chopped almonds

¼ cup chopped green pepper
¼ cup chopped pimentos

Boil 2 cups water with ¼ cup margarine and 1 teaspoon salt. Add above ingredients. Cover and cook over a low heat until rice is fluffy and tender, approximately 40 minutes.

Serves 4

SPANISH RICE

E (*milkless, eggless, glutenless, cornless*)

2 tablespoons milkless margarine
1 cup uncooked rice
8 ounces tomato sauce

½ teaspoon chili powder
½ teaspoon salt
1 cup water

Melt margarine in a large skillet, and brown rice. Add tomato sauce, water, chili powder, and salt, and bring to a boil. Cook 40 minutes if brown rice, or 20 minutes if enriched rice.

Serves 4

RICE AND BROCCOLI

E (*milkless, eggless, glutenless, cornless*)

3 cups cooked rice
2 tablespoons milkless margarine
½ cup chopped onion
1 garlic clove, minced
1 cup sliced mushrooms
½ cup chopped green pepper
1½ pounds fresh broccoli, cut (use only tender stalks), and cooked until just tender
¼ cup chopped pine nuts or chopped almonds
¼ cup chopped parsley

½ cup non-dairy creamer (cornless variety, see Appendix A under *Milk*)
1 teaspoon salt
1 teaspoon thyme
½ teaspoon oregano

In a 10-inch skillet, melt margarine, and sauté onion, garlic, mushrooms, and green pepper until tender. Add cooked broccoli, pine nuts, and rice, and warm through. Stir in creamer. Serve sprinkled with parsley.

Serves 4

SPINACH RICE MOLD

E (*milkless, eggless, glutenless, cornless*)

1 ten-ounce package frozen chopped spinach
3 cups cooked rice
½ teaspoon salt
Dash paprika

Cook spinach per package instructions. Drain and dry with paper towel. Combine spinach, cooked rice, and paprika in a mixing bowl and mix well. Spoon into a greased 4-cup ring mold. Let stand 5 minutes in mold. To unmold, cover ring mold with a serving platter, turn both over together, shake gently, and lift off mold.

Serves 6

ALMONDS AND WILD RICE

E (*milkless, eggless, glutenless, cornless*)

1 cup wild rice, rinsed twice
4 tablespoons milkless margarine
½ cup chopped celery
½ cup slivered almonds
½ cup chopped mushrooms
¼ cup chopped shallots
2 cups Chicken Stock*

In a large skillet, sauté wild rice in margarine until lightly brown. Add celery, almonds, mushrooms and shallots. Sauté until tender, about 5 minutes. Add chicken stock, cover and simmer 30–40 minutes until rice is fluffy.

Serves 4

RICE STUFFING

E (*milkless, eggless, glutenless, cornless*)

3 cups cooked rice
1 tablespoon salt
¼–½ cup Chicken Stock*
1 cup chopped celery
½ cup chopped onion
¼ cup milkless margarine
½ package crisp rice cereal (take care that no wheat or corn are in the cereal)
½ cup water chestnuts
½ cup chopped mushrooms

¼ teaspoon thyme
⅛ teaspoon sage
1 teaspoon marjoram
1 teaspoon poultry seasoning

Melt margarine in a skillet, and sauté mushrooms, onions and celery. Cruch rice cereal into coarse crumbs. Mix together seasonings, stock, rice, and water chestnuts. Add rice cereal and mushrooms and mix thoroughly. Stuff into both cavities of a cleaned, drained, and salted turkey.

Stuffs a 10–12 pound turkey

VEGETABLES

ARTICHOKES WITH LIMA BEANS

E (*milkless, eggless, glutenless, cornless*)

1 ten-ounce package frozen
   artichoke hearts
1 ten-ounce package frozen lima
   beans
3 tablespoons milkless margarine
½ cup chopped onion
1 garlic clove, minced

1 cup diced carrots
1 cup chopped celery
½ cup tomato sauce
½ teaspoon salt
¼ teaspoon thyme
   Water

Thaw artichokes and lima beans. In a 10-inch skillet, melt margarine. Add carrots first and sauté for 5 minutes, then add onions, garlic, and celery, and sauté until vegetables are tender. Add tomato sauce, salt, and thyme. Add artichokes and lima beans, and enough water just to cover chokes. Cover and simmer for 20 minutes or until lima beans and artichokes are tender.

Serves 6

STUFFED ARTICHOKES

E (*milkless, eggless, glutenless, cornless*)

4 large artichokes
1¼ cups dry rice bread* crumbs
⅓ cup freshly grated Romano
   cheese (imported/sheep)

2 tablespoons chopped fresh
   parsley
1 garlic clove, minced (optional)
1 teaspoon salt

[*121*]

Wash and prepare artichokes. Snap spiny tips off outer leaves. In small mixing bowl, mix together bread crumbs, cheese, parsley, garlic, and salt. Push open leaves and spoon mixture into artichoke cavity. Fill two-thirds full. Place stuffed artichokes in an 8-quart saucepan with boiling water 1 to 2 inches deep. Cover and cook 40–50 minutes until leaves are tender.

Serves 4

CARROT AND CAULIFLOWER ROMANO

E (*milkless, eggless, glutenless, cornless*)

6 fresh carrots, cut into strips
1 head of cauliflower
2 cups boiling water
2–3 tablespoons milkless
  margarine

1 clove garlic, minced
2 teaspoons chopped fresh parsley
3 tablespoons freshly grated
  Romano cheese (imported/
  sheep)

Wash, peel, and cut carrots into 2-inch-long strips. Wash cauliflower and separate into flowerets. Place carrots in boiling water, cover, and cook for 7 minutes. Now add cauliflower, and cook another 7 minutes with cover on. Check the vegetables. They should be just done, not overly cooked. Drain.

In an 8–10-inch skillet, melt margarine, and sauté garlic, carrots, and cauliflower over low heat. Remove mixture to a serving dish, and top with fresh parsley and Romano cheese.

Serves 6–8

CARROTS AND MUSHROOMS

E (*milkless, eggless, glutenless, cornless*)

6 carrots, peeled, sliced and
  cooked
1 cup sliced fresh mushrooms
2 tablespoons milkless margarine

½ teaspoon salt
⅛ teaspoon ginger
⅛ teaspoon crushed fennel
½ cup chopped parsley

Cook carrots until just tender. In a skillet, melt margarine, and sauté mushrooms. Add spices, parsley, and cooked carrots. Cover, and simmer until carrots are heated thoroughly.

Serves 4–6

STEWED EGGPLANT

T (*testing for citrus—milkless, eggless, glutenless, cornless*)

2 tablespoons milkless margarine
½ cup chopped onion
1 large eggplant, cut in 1-inch
  cubes
1 teaspoon salt

¼ teaspoon pepper
½ cup water
2 tablespoons lemon juice
  Pinch of allspice

In a skillet, melt margarine, and sauté onion until tender. Add eggplant, salt, pepper, water, lemon juice and allspice. Simmer until tender.

Serves 6

GREEN BEANS ALMONDINE

E (*milkless, eggless, glutenless, cornless*)

1½ pounds fresh green beans
1 quart boiling water
1 cup thinly sliced fresh
  mushrooms

6 tablespoons milkless margarine
½ cup slivered almonds
½ teaspoon garlic salt
  Dash pepper

Sliver beans lengthwise, and place in a large saucepan with boiling water. Cook until beans are just barely tender. Drain and add mushrooms. In separate small saucepan, melt margarine, and brown almonds. Stir in garlic salt and pepper, pour over beans and mushrooms, and heat thoroughly.

Serves 6-8

POTATO BOATS

(*eggless, glutenless, cornless*)

6 medium (6-8 oz.) baking
  potatoes
¼ cup margarine
1 teaspoon salt

¼ teaspoon pepper
½ cup milk, or milk substitute
  (see Appendix A)
  Dash paprika

Wash and dry potatoes; prick skins with a fork; bake about 1 hour at 425° or until tender when pierced. Cutting lengthwise, divide each potato in half. With a spoon, scoop out potato halves to form 12 shells.

In a large bowl, with mixer at low speed, beat potatoes, margarine, salt, and pepper until smooth. Add ¼ cup of milk, beating until smooth. Add remaining milk, if necessary. Spoon mixture back into potato shells, and sprinkle with a dash of paprika. Broil 4–5 minutes, 3 inches from the heat.

Serves 6

NUTTY POTATO BOATS

E (*milkless, eggless, glutenless, cornless*)

8 potatoes
4 ounces Feta cheese (imported/ goat or sheep)
3 tablespoons milkless margarine
3 tablespoons milk substitute (see Appendix A)

¼ cup chopped pine nuts
2 tablespoons grated Romano cheese (imported/sheep)

Scrub potatoes and bake until done. Let cool a little. Cut each potato in half and scoop out all of potato from each skin. Mash potatoes, then add Feta cheese, milk, pine nuts, salt and pepper, and beat with a mixer until smooth. Fill potato jackets with mixture. Sprinkle on Romano cheese, and bake at 350° until cheese is golden brown, about 30 minutes.

Serves 8

FRENCH FRIES

E (*milkless, eggless, glutenless, cornless*)

5 peeled potatoes
1 cup safflower or sesame seed oil
Salt to taste

Thinly slice potatoes, and fry in oil in a hot skillet until lightly browned on both sides. Drain cooked potatoes on paper towel.

Serves 4–6

HASH BROWN POTATOES

E (*milkless, eggless, glutenless, cornless*)

3 medium potatoes, peeled
½ cup chopped onion
¼ cup chopped green peppers

1 teaspoon salt
¼ cup milkless margarine

Cook whole potatoes in boiling water until just tender. Do not overcook. Drain and cool; chop potatoes. Melt margarine in a skillet, and sauté onions and green peppers. Add potatoes; cook until potatoes are just lightly brown. Serve hot.

Serves 4

POTATOES AU GRATIN

E (*milkless, eggless, glutenless, cornless*)

5 medium potatoes
½ cup chopped onions
2 tablespoons milkless margarine
1 cup milk substitute (see Appendix A)

1 teaspoon salt
½ teaspoon paprika
½ cup rice bread* crumbs
2 tablespoons arrowroot flour

In boiling water, cook whole potatoes until just tender. Do not overcook. Melt margarine in a saucepan. Slowly add flour. Stir in salt, paprika, and milk substitute. Drain, cool, and peel and slice potatoes. In a greased 1½-quart casserole dish, place a layer of potatoes then a layer of the sauce mixture. Repeat. Top with bread crumbs, and bake at 350° for 30–40 minutes.

Serves 4–6

POTATO CROQUETTES

(*milkless, glutenless, cornless*)

2 pounds potatoes, peeled and cut into bite-size pieces
⅓ cup freshly grated Romano cheese (imported/sheep)
4 eggs (or substitute, see Appendix A)

1 teaspoon salt
1½ cups chopped fresh parsley
½ cup pine nuts
Potato flour
¾ cup rice bread* crumbs
3–4 tablespoons safflower oil

[*125*]

In an 8-quart saucepan, boil potatoes until tender. Drain and mash well. Turn down the heat and leave mashed potatoes on heat for 5 minutes. Remove from heat, add cheese, 2 eggs, salt, parsley, and pine nuts. Cool. When mixture is cool enough to handle, flour hands with potato flour and roll mashed mixture into rolls 2–3 inches in length, and 1 inch in diameter. Lay them aside on a platter.

In a separate bowl, beat other eggs (or substitute) and in another bowl place bread crumbs. Dunk potato rolls first into egg mixture, then into bread crumb mixture. Place in a 10-inch skillet with oil on medium high heat. Fry until golden brown. Place croquettes on paper towel to drain. Serve immediately or reheat in oven.

Serves 6–8

POTATO PANCAKES

(*milkless, glutenless, cornless*)

4 medium potatoes	1 tablespoon potato flour
2 tablespoons grated onion	2 eggs, well beaten
1 teaspoon salt	5 tablespoons oil
⅛ teaspoon white pepper	

Peel potatoes and soak 1 hour in water. Grate potatoes, and press them in a cheesecloth to drain all liquid out. Add onion, salt, pepper, and flour and mix well. Drop by spoonfuls onto a hot skillet with oil. Fry on both sides until golden brown.

Serves 4

POTATOES WITH PESTO

E (*milkless, eggless, glutenless, cornless*)

4 potatoes (baking potatoes in their skins)	½ cup fresh Basil Pesto*

Wash potatoes and bake them in jackets until tender. When ready to serve, slit and squeeze potato to open. Put a tablespoon of pesto in each potato.

Serves 4

POTATOES WITH PARSLEY SAUCE

E (*milkless, eggless, glutenless, cornless*)

4 tablespoons olive oil
5 boiling potatoes, peeled and sliced
1 clove of garlic, minced
½ cup chopped onions
¼ cup chopped fresh parsley
¼ cup chopped pine nuts
1 teaspoon salt

⅛ teaspoon ground pepper
1¼ cups Chicken Stock* boiling

In a 10-inch skillet, heat olive oil. Add potatoes, and cook over medium high heat until they are golden brown. Add garlic and onion and sauté until tender. Drain excess oil. Add parsley, pine nuts, salt, and pepper. Pour in chicken stock. Cover skillet and simmer over low heat for 25 minutes until potatoes are tender. Transfer them to a platter, and pour the cooking liquid over them.

Serves 4

SALMON-STUFFED POTATOES

(*glutenless, cornless*)

6 russet potatoes
1 (7¾ ounce) can salmon, drained and flaked
¼ cup milk (or substitute, see Appendix A)
1 egg, beaten (or substitute, see Appendix A)
2 tablespoons margarine

¼ cup freshly grated Romano cheese (imported/sheep)
¼ cup sliced shallots

Wash potatoes, and bake them at 400° for 1 hour or until tender. Cut each potato in half lengthwise. Scoop out potato, leaving shell intact. Mash potatoes; add milk, egg, margarine, cheese, and pepper. Add salmon and mix well. Spoon mixture back into shells. Top with shallots, and bake at 375° for 20 minutes or until filling is golden.

Serves 6

POTATO SOUFFLÉ

(*milkless, glutenless, cornless*)

5 tablespoons grated Romano
  cheese (imported/sheep)
2 cups freshly mashed potatoes
1 teaspoon salt
¼ teaspoon pepper
⅛ teaspoon nutmeg
½ cup soy milk, boiling
4 eggs, separated

Preheat oven to 325°. Grease a 6-cup soufflé dish, and sprinkle with 2 tablespoons of the cheese, coating the bottom and sides; tap out any excess.

In a large bowl, combine potatoes, salt, pepper, and nutmeg. Blend in soy milk until smooth. Stir in remaining cheese. Add egg yolks one at a time, beating after each addition. Beat egg whites until stiff but not dry. Stir one-fourth of egg whites into potato mixture; gently fold in rest of whites. Pour mixture into prepared soufflé dish, and smooth out top. Place dish into a baking pan. Pour enough water to reach ½ inch up the side of the dish.

Bake in center of oven for 1½ hours, or until potatoes are golden brown.

Serves 4

SWEET POTATO BALLS

E (*milkless, eggless, glutenless, cornless*)

6 fresh yams or 2 seventeen-ounce
  cans sweet potatoes (with no
  corn syrup)
¼ cup melted milkless margarine
2 tablespoons pure Maple Syrup*
½ teaspoon salt
⅛ teaspoon pepper

Mash peeled yams or sweet potatoes in a large bowl. With mixer at low speed, mix potatoes, margarine, 1 tablespoon maple syrup, salt, and pepper. Mixture should be smooth but stiff. Roll into balls and place into a casserole dish. Spoon remaining syrup over balls. Bake 20 minutes at 350°.

Serves 6–8

SAUTÉED MUSHROOM CAPS

E (*milkless, eggless, glutenless, cornless*)

3 cups whole mushrooms,
   cleaned, with stems chopped off
6 tablespoons milkless margarine
¼ cup chopped shallots
   Salt and pepper to taste

In a saucepan, melt margarine. Add mushroom caps, shallots, salt, and pepper, and cook until just tender.

Serves 4–6

FRESH SPINACH WITH ALMONDS AND PINE NUTS

E (*milkless, eggless, glutenless, cornless*)

3 tablespoons olive oil
1 garlic clove, minced
¼ cup pine nuts
¼ cup almonds, blanched and
   slivered
1 pound freshly cooked spinach,
   drained
1 teaspoon salt

In a large 10-inch skillet, heat olive oil, and sauté garlic for 1 minute. Add pine nuts and almonds, and cook 2 minutes. Add spinach and mix well with nuts. Cook until spinach is heated thoroughly.

Serves 4

SPINACH DUMPLINGS

(milkless, glutenless, cornless)

1 ten-ounce package frozen
  spinach, thawed, chopped, and
  drained in cheesecloth
2 eggs (or substitute, see
  Appendix A)
1 cup rice bread* crumbs
8 ounces tofu, mashed
¼ cup freshly grated Romano
  cheese (imported/sheep)
2 tablespoons chopped onion
1 garlic clove, minced

1 tablespoon chopped parsley
1 teaspoon salt
2 tablespoons potato flour

In a large mixing bowl, combine spinach, eggs (or substitute), bread crumbs, tofu, cheese, onion, garlic, parsley, and salt and mix well. Roll mixture into balls, then roll balls in the flour. In a large saucepan bring to boil 3 cups of water. Add some of the balls; cook until they float to the surface, or 5 minutes. Remove with a slotted spoon to a warm platter. Add remaining balls. Serve hot. This dish is an excellent addition to any stew, spaghetti dish, or just as an appetizer.

Serves 6

BAKED SQUASH

E *(milkless, eggless, glutenless, cornless)*

1 medium acorn, sultan,
  yellow, summer or spaghetti
  squash
3 tablespoons milkless margarine
  Salt and pepper to taste

Preheat oven to 350°. Prepare squash; cut into halves or quarters, and remove seeds. Place squash skin side down on a baking dish. Dot with margarine and bake for 30 minutes until tender.

Serves 4

STUFFED TOMATOES

E (*milkless, eggless, glutenless, cornless*)

6 large tomatoes
1 envelope unflavored gelatin
¼ cup cold Chicken Stock*
2 large cucumbers
1 cup non-dairy creamer (cornless)
½ teaspoon salt
1 teaspoon basil leaves
¼ teaspoon pepper

Soften gelatin in chicken broth. Stir over hot water until gelatin dissolves; cool slightly. Peel and slice cucumbers; finely chop them in a blender or food processor. Put the cucumbers in a mixing bowl and stir in non-dairy creamer, salt, basil leaves, and pepper. Add cooled gelatin and mix thoroughly. Let mixture set. Cut each tomato vertically into 6 sections, almost but not quite to the bottom. Place each tomato on a bed of lettuce, and scoop some of the cucumber gelatin mixture into each tomato.

Serves 6

BAKED STUFFED TOMATOES

E (*milkless, eggless, glutenless, cornless*)

8 large tomatoes, cut in half
2 tablespoons milkless margarine
½ cup chopped shallots
1 garlic clove, minced
¼ cup chopped parsley
½ teaspoon thyme
⅛ teaspoon oregano
½ cup soft rice bread* crumbs
½ teaspoon salt
⅛ teaspoon pepper
¼ cup chopped pine nuts

Wash tomatoes and cut them in half. Scoop out centers and place in a medium-size mixing bowl. In a small skillet, melt margarine, and sauté shallots and garlic until tender. Add shallots and garlic to mixing bowl. Then add parsley, thyme, oregano, bread crumbs, salt, pepper, and pine nuts, and mix ingredients well. Spoon some mixture into each tomato half. Place each stuffed tomato in a lightly greased baking pan. Bake at 425° for 8–10 minutes or until tomatoes are softened.

Serves 8

STIR-FRIED VEGETABLES

T (*testing for alcohol—milkless, eggless, glutenless, cornless*)

2 tablespoons tamari (traditional/ wheat-free)
¼ cup dry sherry
¼ teaspoon salt
¼ teaspoon ground ginger
¼ cup Beef or Chicken Stock*
2 tablespoons safflower oil or soybean oil
1 tablespoon sesame oil

2 garlic cloves, minced
6 cups assorted cut vegetables, washed and thoroughly dried
¼ cup chopped or sliced almonds, if desired

Combine tamari, sherry, salt, ginger, and stock in small bowl. Set aside. Combine the two oils. Preheat a wok or large skillet to medium high heat. When hot, add 1½ tablespoons oil and some minced garlic. Then add another 1½ tablespoons oil and the remaining garlic. First add slow cooking vegetables like carrots, green beans, and broccoli. Turn and flip the vegetables in the hot oil. Then add green peppers, asparagus, celery, and Chinese pea pods, continuing to rapidly stir. Fast cooking vegetables like cabbage, mushrooms, green onions, bean sprouts, and zucchini can be added toward the end of the cooking time. Tomatoes, water chestnuts, bamboo shoots need only to be warmed. Serve vegetables at once with the tamari on the side.

Serves 8

RATATOUILLE

E (*milkless, eggless, glutenless, cornless*)

4 medium tomatoes
1 medium eggplant
4 tablespoons olive oil
1 garlic clove, minced
1 large onion, sliced
2 zucchini, sliced
1 large sweet green pepper, cut into strips
1 large red pepper, cut into strips

1 teaspoon dried basil
1 teaspoon salt
Freshly ground pepper
2 tablespoons chopped fresh parsley

Place tomatoes in boiling water for 10 seconds. Peel and chop roughly. Cut unpeeled eggplant into 1-inch slices. In a large skillet, heat olive oil, add garlic and onion, and sauté until tender. Add eggplant, zucchini, and peppers. Fry vegetables gently. (It may be necessary to add more oil.) Stir in basil, salt, and pepper. Cover and simmer for 30 minutes. Remove lid, add tomatoes and allow them to heat through. Sprinkle with chopped parsley and serve.

Serves 6–8

GRILLED CHEESY ZUCCHINI

E (*milkless, eggless, glutenless, cornless*)

3 tablespoons milkless margarine
1 garlic clove, minced
6 small zucchini, sliced
3 tablespoons chopped fresh parsley
½ teaspoon salt
⅛ teaspoon white pepper
6 ounces Feta cheese (imported/goat), cubed
1½ tablespoons grated Romano cheese (imported/sheep)
3 tablespoons chopped pimento

In a large skillet, melt margarine, and sauté garlic. Add zucchini, cook until tender, then place on a greased cookie sheet. Sprinkle with parsley, salt, and pepper. Top with cubed Feta and grated Romano. Place under broiler for 2 minutes until lightly browned.

Serves 6–8

SKILLET ZUCCHINI

T (*testing for milk—eggless, glutenless, cornless*)

4 small zucchini
4 tablespoons margarine
1 garlic clove, minced
Salt and pepper to taste
1 tablespoon paprika
¼ cup freshly grated Parmesan cheese

Wash and slice zucchini. Melt margarine in a skillet, and sauté garlic and zucchini. When zucchini is just tender, sprinkle with paprika and Parmesan cheese. Serve hot.

Serves 6

SALADS

ARTICHOKE-SPINACH SALAD

E (*milkless, eggless, glutenless, cornless*)

1 eight-ounce artichoke hearts, or
1 nine-ounce package frozen
hearts, chopped
1 cup pitted sliced olives
½ teaspoon salt
¼ teaspoon pepper
½ teaspoon Italian seasoning

1 fifteen-ounce can garbanzo
beans
¼ cup sliced shallots
¼ cup pine nuts
½–1 cup French Dressing II*
Crisp clean romaine lettuce
Crisp clean fresh spinach leaves

Mix above ingredients together, then pour salad dressing over all and mix well.

Serves 4

BEET SALAD

E (*milkless, eggless, glutenless, cornless*)

½ cup sliced beets
¼ cup sliced green onions
½ cup sliced celery
¼ cup sesame seeds

¼ cup garbanzo beans
Eggless Mayonnaise I*
(or see Appendix A)
¼ teaspoon salt
Dash pepper

Mix ingredients together and chill. Serve on a bed of lettuce.

Serves 4

CARROT-RAISIN SALAD

E (*milkless, eggless, glutenless, cornless*)

2 cups shredded carrots
1 cup raisins
½–1 cup Eggless Mayonnaise I*
    (or see Appendix A)
⅓ cup honey (optional)

Mix all ingredients together and refrigerate for at least 1 hour.
Serves 4

AVOCADO SALAD

T (*testing for citrus—milkless, eggless, glutenless, cornless*)

2 avocados, peeled, seeded, and
  sliced
½ pound fresh mushrooms,
  chopped
½ cup chopped water chestnuts
2 tablespoons lemon juice
  French Dressing II*

Mix ingredients together, pour dressing over all, toss and refrigerate. Serve
on a bed of lettuce.
Serves 4

NUTTY FRUIT SALAD

E (*milkless, eggless, glutenless, cornless*)

½ cup chopped blanched almonds
½ cup pitted cherries
½ cup peaches, cut up
½ cup fresh or frozen cranberries,
  cooked
⅓ cup honey
⅓ cup Eggless Mayonnaise I*
  (or see Appendix A)

Combine above ingredients in a mixing bowl. Toss and chill. Serve plain
or on any variety of lettuce leaves.
Serves 4

AVOCADO PROVENÇAL SALAD

E (*milkless, eggless, glutenless, cornless*)

2 heads iceberg lettuce
4 cups fresh spinach
2 cans sliced ripe olives
2 cans artichoke hearts
1 avocado, peeled, pitted, and diced

½ cup sliced shallots
½ cup Curried Italian Dressing*
2 tablespoons chopped parsley

Wash and dry lettuce. Chop greens into bite-size pieces. Chill. In a medium-size bowl, mix olives, artichoke hearts, avocado, shallots, salad dressing, and parsley. Chill for 2 hours. To serve, toss avocado mixture and greens together.

Serves 6–8

BANANA-APPLE SALAD

(*milkless, eggless, glutenless, cornless*)

4 apples (yellow or red), cored, peeled, and cut into bite-size pieces
3 bananas, sliced

½ cup chopped, sliced almonds Eggless Mayonnaise* (or see Appendix A)
¼ cup honey
1 tablespoon lemon juice

Mix above ingredients together. Serve on lettuce leaves, well chilled.

Serves 4

BANANA FRUIT MOLD

(*eggless, glutenless*)

2 three-ounce packages strawberry Jell-O
2 cans crushed pineapple, with juice

1 package frozen strawberries
3 large ripe bananas, mashed
1 cup dairy sour cream (or non-dairy creamer)

[*137*]

Dissolve strawberry Jell-O in 2 cups of boiling water. Stir in pineapple with juice, thawed berries, and mashed bananas. Stir to blend evenly. Pour half of mixture into a large greased tube mold. Place in refrigerator until firm. Lightly whip sour cream (or non-dairy creamer) with a whisk. Spread over the firm gelatin layer. Pour remaining half of mixture over layer of sour cream. Return to refrigerator for several hours, or until firm enough to cut.

Serves 12

BEAN SALAD SUPREME

(*milkless, eggless, glutenless, cornless*)

1 sixteen-ounce can garbanzo beans
1 sixteen-ounce can red kidney beans
1 sixteen-ounce can lima beans
½ pound French beans, cooked and sliced
½ cup chopped shallots

4 medium tomatoes, chopped
¼ cup finely chopped green pepper
¼ cup chopped celery
¼ cup blanched almonds, chopped
2 tablespoons lemon juice
Salt and pepper to taste
Assorted lettuce
Sprig of watercress for garnish

Place garbanzo beans, kidney beans, lima beans, French beans, shallots, tomatoes, peppers, and celery in a large mixing bowl. Sprinkle with almonds, lemon juice, salt, and pepper. Toss and chill at least 1 hour. Serve on a bed of lettuce and garnish with watercress.

Serves 6–8

CHINESE CHICKEN SALAD

E (*milkless, eggless, glutenless, cornless*)

3 cups cooked chicken
3 handfuls mai fun (rice sticks)
¼ cup sliced scallions
½ cup chopped Chinese parsley
1 head iceberg lettuce

Dressing:
½ teaspoon dry mustard
2 teaspoons sugar

1½ teaspoons tamari (traditional/ wheat-free)
1 teaspoon sesame oil
⅓ cup safflower oil
3 tablespoons Chinese rice vinegar

Shred with fingers enough cooked chicken for 3 cups. Fry rice sticks (mai fun) according to package directions. Place sliced iceberg lettuce on a platter, top with chicken, sliced scallions, chopped parsley and crisp mai fun.

Mix dressing in a separate bowl with a whisk. Pour over salad, and serve immediately.

Serves 4

CRANBERRY APPLE MOLD

E (*milkless, eggless, glutenless, cornless*)

2 envelopes unflavored gelatin	2 apples, seeded and chopped
½ cup cold water	2 cups chopped celery
2½ cups apple juice	2½ cups chopped almonds
2 cups ground raw cranberries	½ cup sugar

Soften gelatin in cold water and dissolve over low heat. Remove from heat and stir in apple juice. Chill until partially set. Combine cranberries, apples, celery, almonds, and sugar. Add cranberry-almond mixture to partially set gelatin and pour into a mold. Chill until firm.

Serves 6

CUCUMBER SALAD PLATTER

E (*milkless, eggless, glutenless, cornless*)

2 large cucumbers, sliced	2 tablespoons olive oil
4 large tomatoes, sliced	2 tablespoons wine vinegar
2 fifteen-ounce cans pitted olives, drained	Salt and pepper to taste
	¼ teaspoon oregano
1 small onion, finely chopped	1 clove garlic, minced

Prepare cucumbers, tomatoes, and olives. Place in a casserole dish. In a small mixing bowl, mix together onions, oil, wine vinegar, oregano, garlic, salt, and pepper. Pour dressing over vegetables, and marinate 2–3 hours before serving.

Serves 4

FETA SALAD

E (*milkless, eggless, glutenless, cornless*)

1 medium eggplant
1 cup chopped onions
4 tablespoons olive oil
2 tablespoons vinegar
½ teaspoon salt
⅛ teaspoon pepper
¼ cup chopped parsley
3 medium tomatoes, sliced
  Black olives
1 large green pepper, cut into
  strips

4 ounces Feta cheese (imported/
  goat), cubed

Wrap whole eggplant in aluminum foil. Bake in a preheated 350° oven for 35–45 minutes. Peel off skin, and cut eggplant into cubes. In a mixing bowl, combine eggplant with onion, oil, vinegar, salt, and pepper to taste. Chill for 2 hours. To serve, place on a salad platter, sprinkle with parsley, and surround with remaining ingredients.

Serves 8

FRUIT SALAD

(*milkless, eggless, glutenless, cornless*)

1 large cantaloupe, cut into
  bite-size pieces
½ watermelon, cut into bite-size
  pieces
¼ cup raisins
3 apples, cored, peeled, and cubed
2 bananas, sliced
2 peaches, peeled and cut into
  bite-size pieces
½ cup pitted fresh cherries (or
  frozen)

½ pound green grapes, peeled
  (optional)
  Eggless Mayonnaise* (or see
  Appendix A)
¼ cup honey
2 tablespoons lemon juice

Mix ingredients together. Serve chilled.

Serves 6

GARBANZO-KIDNEY BEAN SALAD

E (*milkless, eggless, glutenless, cornless*)

1 sixteen-ounce can garbanzo
  beans
1 sixteen-ounce can red kidney
  beans
½ cup chopped shallots
½ cup chopped celery
1 two-ounce can sliced black
  olives
1 garlic clove, minced
2 tomatoes, cut into wedges
½ cup chopped fresh parsley
¼ cup olive oil

2 tablespoons vinegar
½ teaspoon salt'
  Freshly ground black pepper

Combine all ingredients. Chill for several hours before serving.

Serves 6

GREEK SALAD

E (*milkless, eggless, glutenless, cornless*)

½ pound fresh spinach
½ pound iceberg, or other green
  lettuce
3 large tomatoes, cut into wedges
1 cucumber, peeled and sliced
1 tablespoon capers
¼ cup chopped celery
½ cup fresh mushrooms, sliced

1 can (2½ ounces) black olives,
  sliced
2 slices Feta cheese (imported/
  goat or sheep)

Wash fresh spinach and iceberg lettuce. Pat dry with paper towel. Tear into bite-size strips and lay on a platter. Combine other ingredients, except for cheese, in a mixing bowl, then pour on top of lettuce. Crush Feta and sprinkle it on top of salad. Top with Greek Salad Dressing*.

Serves 4–6

GREEN SALAD

E (*milkless, eggless, glutenless, cornless*)

Any combination of crisp lettuce, cleaned and dried

½ cup chopped scallions
½ cup sliced cucumbers

¼ cup chopped radishes
2 tomatoes, wedged (optional)

Prepare bed of lettuce. Place scallions, cucumbers, radishes, and tomatoes on top. Serve with salad dressing of choice.

Serves 4

MUSHROOM-CUCUMBER SALAD

E (*milkless, eggless, glutenless, cornless*)

¼ pound sliced fresh mushrooms
1 cucumber, peeled and sliced
¼ cup sliced shallots

½ cup frozen peas, thawed
¼ cup chopped celery
Assorted greens

Serve salad with dressing of choice.

ORIENTAL SPINACH-SESAME SALAD

(*milkless, eggless, glutenless, cornless*)

1 bunch fresh spinach
¼ cup sesame seeds
2 tablespoons safflower oil
2 tablespoons lemon juice
2 tablespoons tamari (traditional/ wheat-free)

1 teaspoon salt
⅛ teaspoon hot pepper sauce
1 cup fresh mushrooms, thinly sliced
1 can water chestnuts, drained and sliced

Rinse spinach leaves and drain well. Tear into bite-size pieces, and chill. In a medium-size saucepan, heat sesame seeds until brown. Add oil, lemon juice, tamari, salt, and hot pepper sauce. Pour mixture into a salad bowl. Chill for at least 1 hour. Before serving, add spinach leaves and toss well.

Serves 4

PACHADI

T (*testing for corn—milkless, eggless, glutenless*)

1 cup shredded green cabbage
1 cup grated carrots
1 cup unpeeled sliced cucumber
2 green chili peppers, cut in slivers
1 cup chopped shallots
1 teaspoon tamari (traditional/ wheat-free)

1 cup non-dairy whipped topping (contains corn syrup)
½ teaspoon paprika
1 tablespoon ground coriander or chopped watercress sprigs

Combine all ingredients except watercress. Chill for 2 hours. When serving, garnish with watercress.

Serves 4

POTATO SALAD

E (*milkless, eggless, glutenless, cornless*)

5 medium potatoes, peeled, washed, and diced
1 tablespoon salt
½ teaspoon paprika
1 cup diced celery
½ cup diced green pepper
½ cup chopped dill pickles

2 tablespoons chopped parsley
½ cup sliced scallions
1½ tablespoons prepared mustard
1–1½ cups Eggless Mayonnaise I* (or see Appendix A)
½ cup chopped onion

Cook potatoes until tender, then drain for approximately 15 minutes. Add other ingredients and mix well. Refrigerate 2 hours before serving.

Serves 6

ROQUEFORT AND TOMATO SALAD

E (*milkless, eggless, glutenless, cornless*)

1 tablespoon red wine vinegar
3 tablespoons olive oil
½ teaspoon salt

3 medium tomatoes, chopped
2 tablespoons Roquefort Cheese

Mix together the vinegar, oil, salt, and pepper and pour over tomatoes. Let chill 1 hour, then sprinkle with cheese. Serve on a bed of lettuce.

Serves 4

APPLE NUT SLAW

(*milkless, eggless, glutenless, cornless*)

3 cups unpeeled red apples, cored and chopped
1 cup pine nuts
4 cups shredded green cabbage
1 cup non-dairy whipped topping (cornless)
2 tablespoons lemon juice
1 tablespoon honey

1 teaspoon salt
¼ teaspoon pepper

In a large bowl, combine all ingredients. Chill for 1 hour before serving.

Serves 4

TABBOULÉH

T (*testing for gluten—milkless, eggless, cornless*)

¼ cup cracked wheat (bulgur)
1 bunch scallions, sliced
½ cup chopped fresh parsley
3 tablespoons dried mint

3–4 large tomatoes, cut into wedges
Salt and pepper to taste
Cayenne to taste
2–3 tablespoons olive oil

Soak cracked wheat in water for ½ hour. Drain and squeeze out as much moisture as possible. Spread out to dry until ready to use. In a large mixing bowl, place scallions, parsley, and mint. Add tomatoes and toss with other vegetables. Add cracked wheat and mix well. Add remaining ingredients, toss salad, and place on beds of romaine lettuce.

Serves 4–6

TURKEY SALAD

E (*milkless, eggless, glutenless, cornless*)

2 cups diced, cooked turkey meat
1 cup sliced fresh mushrooms
1 cup peeled, sliced cucumbers
½ cup chopped water chestnuts
½ cup sliced scallions
1 teaspoon basil
½–1 cup Eggless Mayonnaise I* (or see
    Appendix A)
½ cup sliced almonds
    Crisp lettuce, washed and dried
    Ground pepper

Pour lemon juice over cleaned and sliced mushrooms, then mix them with
other ingredients. Refrigerate the salad for at least 1 hour. Serve on crisp
lettuce with ground pepper to taste.

Serves 4

WALDORF SALAD

(*milkless, eggless, glutenless, cornless*)

½ non-dairy creamer (cornless
    variety, see Appendix A under
    Milk)
1 tablespoon honey
1 tablespoon lemon juice
¼ cup Eggless Mayonnaise* (or see
    Appendix A)
3½ cups diced apples, unpeeled
1¼ cups chopped celery
¾ cup chopped walnuts

Whisk together creamer, honey, lemon juice, and mayonnaise in a large
salad bowl. Chill. Core and dice unpeeled apples. Add apples, celery, and
walnuts to chilled dressing in salad bowl. Toss well.

Serves 4

ZUCCHINI SALAD

T (*testing for egg—milkless, glutenless, cornless*)

2 small zucchini, sliced
2 large tomatoes, cut into wedges
¼ head iceberg lettuce, shredded
¼ head romaine lettuce, chopped
½ cup chopped shallots
2 tablespoons chopped parsley

1 two-ounce jar pimento, chopped
1 hard-boiled egg, chopped
1 garlic clove, minced
½ cup sesame seed oil
Salt

Brush zucchini slices with oil, place them on a cookie sheet and broil until lightly browned. Dice cooked zucchini and add lettuces, shallots, parsley, and pimento; toss. Whisk garlic, lemon juice, and sesame seed oil together to make dressing. When ready to serve, place on a platter, garnish with diced egg and pour on dressing.

Serves 4–6

DRESSINGS AND SAUCES

FRENCH DRESSING I

E (*milkless, eggless, glutenless, cornless*)

1½ cups safflower oil
½ cup tarragon vinegar
1 teaspoon salt

½ teaspoon pepper
2 teaspoons chopped shallots
1 teaspoon paprika

Mix ingredients and refrigerate 2 days before using.

Makes 2 cups

FRENCH DRESSING II

E (*milkless, eggless, glutenless, cornless*)

1 cup safflower or olive oil
2 tablespoons paprika
1 clove garlic, minced
¼ cup vinegar

1 teaspoon salt
2 tablespoons chopped fresh
  parsley
Dash cayenne pepper

Combine all above ingredients, mix well with a whisk, and refrigerate.

Makes 1½ cups

ROQUEFORT DRESSING I

E (*milkless, eggless, glutenless, cornless*)

4 ounces Roquefort cheese
  (imported/sheep)
⅛ teaspoon ground pepper
2 tablespoons minced onion
¼ teaspoon paprika

1 teaspoon honey
1 garlic clove, minced
⅓ cup wine vinegar
¼ cup olive oil

Combine ingredients with a mixing whisk and refrigerate.

Makes 2 cups

ROQUEFORT DRESSING II

E (*milkless, eggless, glutenless, cornless*)

1 cup Eggless Mayonnaise I*
  (or see Appendix A)
⅓ cup milk substitute (see
  Appendix A)
¼ cup Roquefort cheese
  (imported/sheep)

1 garlic clove, minced
3 tablespoons vinegar
  Cayenne pepper

Combine ingredients with a mixing whisk and refrigerate.

Makes 1½ cups

VINAIGRETTE DRESSING

(*milkless, glutenless, cornless*)

2 tablespoons French Dressing II
  (above)
1½ cups olive oil
½ cup vinegar

4 tablespoons finely chopped dill
  pickles
4 tablespoons chopped chives
1 hard-cooked egg, chopped

Combine oil and vinegar and mix with a whisk. Add remaining ingredients and mix well.

Makes 2 cups

DILLWEED SAUCE

(milkless, eggless, glutenless, cornless)

1 medium dill pickle, finely
   chopped
1 teaspoon dill weed
½ teaspoon salt

⅛ teaspoon pepper
1 tablespoon lemon juice
1 tablespoon snipped chives
¼ cup milkless margarine

Melt margarine in a saucepan. Add lemon juice, chives, salt, pepper, and dill weed; mix well. Add chopped pickles before serving.

Makes ½ cup

ITALIAN-STYLE ROQUEFORT DRESSING

E *(milkless, eggless, glutenless, cornless)*

1 pint French Dressing II*
1 garlic clove, minced

4 ounces Roquefort cheese,
   crumbled (imported/sheep)
3 tablespoons non-dairy creamer
   (cornless)

Combine all ingredients with a whisk. Store in refrigerator.

Makes 1½ pints

EGGLESS MAYONNAISE I

E *(milkless, eggless, glutenless, cornless)*

1 tablespoon arrowroot flour or
   potato flour
1 teaspoon salt
½ teaspoon paprika
3 tablespoons vinegar

1 cup cold water
1 teaspoon Dijon-type mustard
Pinch Tabasco
2 cups olive oil

Dissolve flour, salt, paprika and vinegar in water. Place in a double boiler and cook until mixture thickens, stirring quite often. Cook an additional 2 minutes. Add mustard and Tabasco. Add oil 1 teaspoon at a time, beating constantly. Store in refrigerator.

Makes 2 cups

EGGLESS MAYONNAISE II

(*milkless, eggless, glutenless, cornless*)

1 teaspoon sugar
1 teaspoon salt
⅓ teaspoon paprika
1 teaspoon dry mustard
¼ cup canned milk substitute (see Appendix A)

⅓ cup safflower oil
3 teaspoons vinegar
3 teaspoons lemon juice
⅔ cup safflower oil

Mix together sugar, salt, paprika, and dry mustard. Add milk substitute. Add ⅓ cup salad oil 1 teaspoon at a time, and beat well. In a separate bowl, mix together vinegar and lemon juice. Add this mixture alternately with ⅔ cup salad oil. Mix well after each addition. Cover and chill.

Makes 1¼ cups

TARRAGON DRESSING

E (*milkless, eggless, glutenless, cornless*)

½ cup tarragon vinegar
1 cup olive oil
1 teaspoon Dijon-type mustard

¼ cup chopped shallots
½ teaspoon ground pepper
1 teaspoon salt

Combine above ingredients with a whisk and refrigerate.

Makes 1½ cups

GREEK SALAD DRESSING

E (*milkless, eggless, glutenless, cornless*)

½ cup wine vinegar
½ teaspoon oregano
1 teaspoon Dijon-type mustard
½ teaspoon crumbled bay leaf

1 cup olive oil
⅛ teaspoon ground pepper
2 tablespoons grated onion
½ teaspoon salt

Combine above ingredients with a whisk and refrigerate.

Makes 1½ cups

CURRIED ITALIAN DRESSING

E (*milkless, eggless, glutenless, cornless*)

1 tablespoon Italian seasoning
(see Ingredient Glossary under
Herbs and Spices)
4 tablespoons red wine vinegar
2 tablespoons minced parsley
½ teaspoon curry powder

2 tablespoons Dijon-type mustard
½ cup safflower oil or olive oil
¼ teaspoon salt
⅛ teaspoon pepper
Dash garlic powder

Combine above ingredients in a small bowl. Chill.

Makes ¾ cup

TAHINI SAUCE

(*milkless, eggless, cornless*)

1 cup sesame paste
¼ cup cold water
2 tablespoons lemon juice
2 tablespoons minced parsley

1 garlic clove, minced
½ teaspoon salt
⅛ teaspoon pepper

Mix ingredients together in a mixing bowl with a whisk. Store in refrigerator, sealed.

Makes 1¼ cups

WHITE SAUCE I

E (*milkless, eggless, glutenless, cornless*)

¼ cup milkless margarine
1 tablespoon potato flour
2 tablespoons tapioca flour

1 cup milk substitute (see
Appendix A)
1 teaspoon salt
¼ teaspoon pepper

Melt margarine in a saucepan. Add tapioca flour slowly, then potato flour. Gradually pour in milk, stirring constantly until sauce is thickened. Season with salt and pepper.

Makes 1 cup

WHITE SAUCE II

E (*milkless, eggless, glutenless, cornless*)

¼ cup milkless margarine
3 tablespoons arrowroot flour
1 cup milk substitute (see
   Appendix A)

1 teaspoon salt
¼ teaspoon pepper

Melt margarine in a saucepan. Add arrowroot flour slowly. Gradually pour in milk, stirring constantly. Season with salt and pepper.

Makes 1 cup

MUSTARD SAUCE

E (*milkless, eggless, glutenless, cornless*)

2 tablespoons Dijon-type mustard
1 tablespoon honey
2 tablespoons vinegar
6 tablespoons safflower oil

1 tablespoon chopped dill
½ teaspoon fennel seed, chopped
2 tablespoons minced parsley

Mix mustard with honey and vinegar; add oil slowly, beating as you add. Stir in chopped dill, fennel seed, and parsley. Chill.

Makes 1 cup

TARTAR SAUCE

(*milkless, eggless, glutenless, cornless*)

½ cup Eggless Mayonnaise* (or see
   Appendix A)
1 cup chopped dill pickle
3 tablespoons grated onion
2 tablespoons chopped fresh
   parsley

1 tablespoon lemon juice
1 teaspoon tarragon
1 teaspoon finely chopped capers
¼ teaspoon salt
⅛ teaspoon pepper

Combine above ingredients thoroughly with a whisk and chill overnight.

Makes ¾ cup

BÉCHAMEL SAUCE

E (*milkless, eggless, glutenless, cornless*)

4 tablespoons milkless margarine
½ cup finely chopped onions
4 tablespoons tapioca flour
2 tablespoons potato flour
2 cups hot milk substitute (see Appendix A)

¼ cup finely chopped celery
½ teaspoon thyme
¼ teaspoon bay leaf
⅛ teaspoon salt
⅛ teaspoon white pepper
⅛ teaspoon nutmeg

Melt margarine in a large saucepan over low heat. Add onion, and sauté until tender. Add flour and blend in well. Add milk substitute and stir in circle eights. Add remaining ingredients, and stir until thick and creamy.

Makes 2¼ cups

MUSHROOM SAUCE

E (*milkless, eggless, glutenless, cornless*)

2 tablespoons milkless margarine
1 cup mushrooms, chopped
2 tablespoons soy flour

2 cups chicken broth
¼ cup non-dairy creamer (cornless)

In a saucepan, melt margarine, and sauté mushrooms until tender. Stir in soy flour, then slowly add chicken broth. Cover and simmer for 10 minutes until thickened. Remove from heat, and add creamer.

Makes 2½ cups

DRIED MINT

2 bunches fresh mint

Wash and dry mint leaves. Chop the mint and spread on a greased cookie sheet. Place overnight in a gas oven. In an electric oven, bake on warm for 3 hours. Store in an air-tight container.

BOUQUET GARNI

Tie up in cheesecloth:

6 sprigs parsley
8 leaves basil

3 cloves garlic, unpeeled, slightly crushed
1 large bay leaf
7 peppercorns

COCONUT STOCK

1 cup unsweetened coconut

2 cups hot water

Place coconut and hot water in a blender. Blend at high speed for 1 minute. Stop machine and scrape down sides of container with a spatula. Blend again until liquid is thickened. Pour contents through a sieve lined with cheesecloth. Tightly cover and refrigerate.

Makes 2 cups

PREPARED MISO SAUCE

E (*milkless, eggless, glutenless, cornless*)

1 cup water
4 ounces brown rice miso

1 tablespoon tamari (traditional/ wheat-free)

Over low heat, gradually add water to miso and tamari mixture and stir until you have a smooth sauce. Do not overheat. Refrigerate.

NOTE: This mixture also works as a soup.

Makes 1¼ cups

HEADACHE-FREE SEASONED SALT

E (*milkless, eggless, glutenless, cornless*)

4 teaspoons Italian seasoning (see Ingredient Glossary under *Herbs and Spices*)
2 teaspoons tumeric

4 teaspoons garlic salt
4 teaspoons onion salt
2 teaspoons paprika
2 teaspoons potato flour

Mix seasonings. Store in a sealed container.

BREADS, MUFFINS, AND CEREALS

When one cooks with flours that contain no gluten, it is necessary to use eggs to achieve any type of texture or structure. However, until the individual is tested for allergy to eggs, this will not be possible. Yeast-raised breads must be used during the elimination diet. Use any of the commercial gluten-free rice bread mixes, following their instructions. Or if yeast is suspected, use a wheatless, milkless, eggless muffin recipe as a substitute for bread. Also, be sure to use a cereal-free, egg-free baking powder when baking powder is called for.

The cook using this diet should also note that a variety of flours are added to recipes with rice flour to add moisture. Soy flour is an excellent addition to a recipe for cakes because it helps retain moisture. Potato flour is also good, yet care should be taken with this flour as too much in a bread or cake will result in a heavy, extremely moist product.

The following chart will show how these flours and others compare to wheat flour.

1 cup wheat flour = 1 cup corn flour
¾ cup potato flour
⅞ cup rice flour
· 1 cup soy flour
1 cup tapioca flour
¾ cup arrowroot flour

RICE PANCAKES

E (*milkless, eggless, glutenless, cornless*)

1 egg substitute (see Appendix A)
¾ cup rice flour
2 tablespoons soy flour
1 tablespoon safflower oil
½ teaspoon salt

½ teaspoon honey
1½ teaspoons baking powder (cereal-free, egg-free)
¾ cup water or milk substitute (see Appendix A)

In a mixing bowl, beat egg substitute. Add flours, powder, and salt, mix well, then add honey and water (or milk substitute). Cook on a hot griddle, using about ¼ cup batter for each pancake. Turn once.

Makes 10–15 pancakes

BASIC ALLERGY-FREE WAFFLES

E (*milkless, eggless, glutenless, cornless*)

By adding 1 tablespoon safflower oil, the batter for Rice Pancakes* can be used to make waffles.

Serves 4

APRICOT NUT BREAD

E (*milkless, eggless, glutenless, cornless*)

¼ cup chopped naturally dried apricots
1 cup rice flour
2 tablespoons soy flour
½ cup sugar
1½ tablespoons baking powder
1 teaspoon baking soda

½ teaspoon salt
1 egg substitute (see Appendix A)
½ cup milk substitute
2 tablespoons milkless margarine
½ cup chopped almonds

Sift together dry ingredients. Set aside. Melt margarine, then slowly add sugar and egg substitute until creamed. Add dry ingredients and milk alternately. Blend in almonds. Pour into a greased loaf pan. Bake 1 hour at 350°.

Makes 1 loaf

EGGLESS COFFEE CAKE

(eggless, cornless)

1 tablespoon margarine, melted
1 cup sugar
½ cup margarine, melted
1 teaspoon vanilla
3 tablespoons safflower oil
3 tablespoons water
2 teaspoons baking powder
  (egg-free)
1⅞ cup flour
2 tablespoons potato starch

1 teaspoon each of baking
  powder and soda
½ teaspoon salt
½ cup ricotta cheese
1 cup milk
Topping:
½ cup ground almonds
¼ cup sugar
⅓ cup brown sugar
1 teaspoon cinnamon
2 tablespoons margarine, softened

Pour 1 tablespoon melted margarine into greased bundt pan. Place half of mixed topping over melted margarine. Cream margarine, sugar and vanilla together. Combine oil, water, and baking soda and add to creamed mixture. Sift dry ingredients together and add to creamed batter, alternating with ricotta and milk. Spread half of the batter over topping in the bundt pan, and top with remaining topping and batter. Bake at 350° for 40–45 minutes.

Serves 8

BANANA LOAF

(milkless, glutenless)

2 cups soy flour
½ cup rice flour (sift 3 times)
1 teaspoon baking soda
1 teaspoon salt
2 teaspoons baking powder
1¼ cups sugar
2 medium bananas, mashed

½ cup milk substitute (see
  Appendix A)
2 eggs (or substitute, see
  Appendix A)
½ teaspoon lemon juice
1 teaspoon vanilla
½ cup milkless margarine

Sift dry ingredients together and set aside. Melt butter, add sugar slowly, creaming well. Add eggs (or substitute), bananas, and vanilla. Mix until smooth. Slowly add milk and lemon juice to banana mixture alternately with flours until well mixed. Pour into a greased loaf pan. Bake at 350° for 75 minutes or until brown. This loaf will *not* spring back upon touch. Therefore, testing for doneness is difficult.

Makes 1 loaf

BANANA NUT BREAD

T (*testing for gluten—eggless, milkless, cornless*)

½ cup milkless margarine
1 cup sugar
2 cups flour

1 teaspoon baking soda
3 bananas, mashed
½ cup chopped nuts

Cream margarine, add sugar and beat until fluffy. Add flour, baking soda, mashed bananas, and lemon juice, and mix until smooth. Stir in nuts. Pour into a greased and floured loaf pan. Bake at 350–375° for 30 to 45 minutes.

Makes 1 loaf

BLUEBERRY MUFFINS

(*milkless, glutenless, cornless*)

1½ cup rice flour
¼ cup potato flour
1 cup washed blueberries
¼ cup milkless margarine
4 tablespoons sugar

1 egg, well beaten (or substitute, see Appendix A)
4 teaspoons baking powder
½ teaspoon salt
1 cup milk substitute (see Appendix A)

Mix sifted flours together twice. Mix ¼ cup of sifted flour with blueberries. Cream margarine and sugar, and add egg. Sift together baking powder, salt and remaining flour. Add the dry ingredients to egg mixture alternately with milk. Add floured berries last. Bake in greased muffin pans for 25 minutes at 425°F.

Makes 10–15 muffins

BLUEBERRY POPOVERS

(*milkless, glutenless, cornless*)

Blueberry mixture:
3 cups brown sugar

1 cup blueberries

Popover mixture:
½ cup potato starch
½ cup soy flour
½ cup sugar
2 tablespoons baking powder
½ teaspoon salt

2 eggs, separated, at room
temperature
½ cup cold water
2 tablespoons milkless margarine
1 tablespoon brown sugar

Mix blueberries and brown sugar together and set aside. Sift dry ingredients twice. Mix egg yolks and water and add to dry ingredients. Stir in melted margarine. In a separate bowl, beat egg whites until stiff but not dry. Mix one quarter of egg whites into flour mixture, then fold in remaining egg whites. Pour batter into a greased muffin pan, filling each tin half full. Spoon 2 tablespoons of blueberry mixture onto each popover, sprinkle brown sugar on top, then top each with another spoonful of popover batter. Bake at 400° for 15–20 minutes.

Makes 8 popovers

CRANBERRY ALMOND BREAD

(*milkless, glutenless, cornless*)

2 cups whole fresh cranberries
1¼ cup rice flour
¼ cup soy flour
⅓ cup potato starch
1 teaspoon baking soda
1 teaspoon cream of tartar
1 teaspoon salt
1 teaspoon vinegar
2 eggs, well beaten (or egg
substitute, see Appendix A)

1¼ cups apple juice
3 tablespoons safflower oil
½ cup almonds, chopped

Wash cranberries, and chop them in a blender or food processor. Sift together the next 6 ingredients twice. In a separate bowl, mix together vinegar, eggs, oil, and apple juice. Combine with flour mixture. Add almonds, and mix well. Fold in chopped cranberries. Pour into a greased and floured loaf pan. Bake at 350° for 60 minutes.

Makes 1 loaf

CRANBERRY PANCAKES

E (*milkless, eggless, glutenless, cornless*)

Use Rice Pancake* recipe, but increase the water or milk to ¾ cup. Pour batter into a pitcher and allow to stand 30 minutes.

½ cup sugar
2 tablespoons milkless margarine
3 cups cooked cranberries, fresh or
   frozen

Dissolve sugar in 1 tablespoon milkless margarine. Add cleaned and drained cranberries. Make pancake batter and set aside. In a small skillet, melt 1 tablespoon margarine and tilt pan to coat sides. Pour ¼ cup batter into pan and tilt pan again to spread batter evenly. Cook for about 1 minute, then add 1 cup of the cranberry mixture. Pour another ¼ cup of batter over cranberries. When bottom pancake is lightly brown turn to brown the other side. When this other side is brown and cranberries cooked, remove from skillet like an omelet. Sprinkle with confectioner's sugar.

Makes 15 pancakes

MOLASSES BREAD

(*milkless, glutenless, cornless*)

2 eggs (or substitute, see
   Appendix A)
2 tablespoons safflower oil
½ cup raisins
⅓ cup honey
⅓ cup molasses
¾ cup very hot water
⅞ cup rice flour
1 cup rice bran

1 tablespoon potato flour
1 teaspoon baking soda
1 teaspoon baking powder
1 teaspoon salt

Sift dry ingredients together and set aside. Cream honey, oil, and eggs (or substitute) together, add molasses; then add hot water and dry ingredients alternately. Add raisins to the batter, then pour into a greased baking pan or loaf pan. Bake at 350° for 1 hour.

Serves 8

RICE LOAF BREAD

E (*milkless, eggless, glutenless, cornless*)

1½ cups brown rice flour
2 tablespoons soy flour
2 tablespoons potato flour
¼ cup rice bran (or rice polish)

2 cups milk substitute (see
   Appendix A)
2 tablespoons safflower oil
2 tablespoons baking powder
2 egg substitutes (see
   Appendix A), mixed

Mix above ingredients together in a mixing bowl, and pour into a greased loaf pan. Bake 1 hour at 350°.

Makes 1 loaf

JOHNNY CAKES

T (*testing for corn—milkless, glutenless*)

½ cup sugar
¼ cup milkless margarine
1 egg, beaten (or egg substitute,
   see Appendix A)
1 cup milk substitute (see
   Appendix A)
1 cup yellow cornmeal

¾ cup rice flour
1 tablespoon potato flour
1 teaspoon salt
1 teaspoon cream of tartar
1 teaspoon baking soda

In a large mixing bowl, cream sugar and margarine together. Add ⅓ cup of milk substitute, reserving the rest for later. In another bowl, mix together flours, salt, cream of tartar, and soda. Add flour mixture to margarine alternately with reserved milk, stirring well after each addition. Bake in an 8 × 8 × 2-inch greased pan in a 350° oven for 30 minutes or until golden brown. Cut into squares to serve.

Serves 8

POLENTA

T (*testing for corn—milkless, eggless, glutenless*)

1 tablespoon salt
1¾ cups coarse-grained cornmeal

5 cups water

In a large, heavy saucepan, bring water to a boil. Add salt, lower heat so water is just simmering. Add cornmeal a little at a time with your hands. With a wooden spoon, stir constantly in a figure eight. Continue stirring for 15–20 minutes after adding cornmeal. When it pulls away from sides of pan, remove polenta to a large wooden board, and shape into a round mold. Serve hot.

Serves 4

FRIED POLENTA

T (*testing for corn—milkless, eggless, glutenless*)

Cooled Polenta*, sliced into ½-inch
  pieces
1 cup vegetable oil

In a large skillet, heat oil until hot. Place slices of polenta into oil, cook until a slight crust forms, then turn over and do other side. Transfer to paper towels to drain.

Serves 4

SOUTHERN SPOON CORN BREAD

(*milkless, glutenless*)

1 cup cornmeal	2 cups milk substitute (see
2 cups boiling water	Appendix A)
1 tablespoon milkless margarine	2½ teaspoons baking powder
2 eggs, well beaten	(cereal-free)
1 teaspoon salt	

Scald cornmeal with water, stir thoroughly, then cool. Add melted margarine, eggs, salt, and milk substitute. Add baking powder. The batter should be quite thin. Pour into a greased baking dish, and bake at 350° for 30–40 minutes. Serve with a spoon from the pan.

Serves 4

SURPRISE CORNBREAD

T (*testing for corn—milkless, glutenless*)

2 eggs (or substitute, see
Appendix A)
¼ cup corn oil
1 two-ounce can green chiles,
seeded and finely chopped
1 small can corn, with liquid
½ cup tofu, mashed

1 cup yellow cornmeal
1 teaspoon salt
2 teaspoons baking powder
2 cups grated Kassari cheese
(imported/sheep)

In a large mixing bowl, beat eggs and oil until well blended. Add chiles, corn, tofu, cornmeal, salt, baking powder and 1½ cups of cheese. Combine and stir until well blended, then pour into a 8 × 8 × 2-inch greased baking dish. Sprinkle with remaining cheese. Bake in 350° oven for 1 hour. Serve hot.

Serves 6

BASIC RICE MUFFINS

(*milkless, glutenless, cornless*)

½ cup rice flour (see Appendix A)
½ cup rice polish (see Appendix A)
2 tablespoons any wheat-free
flour
1 tablespoon safflower oil

1 cup milk substitute (see
Appendix A)
1 egg
1½ teaspoons baking powder

Mix ingredients together. Pour batter into a greased muffin pan. Bake at 425° for 20 minutes.

Any of the following ingredients may be added:

¼ cup raisins
¼ cup chopped almonds
¼ cup chopped dates
¼ cup peeled, cored, and shredded
apples

Makes 8-10 muffins

GARRETT'S CINNAMON MUFFINS

(*milkless, glutenless, cornless*)

Use the batter from the Blueberry Popovers*, but decrease the baking powder to 2 teaspoons and the milkless margarine to 1 tablespoon.

½ cup brown sugar
2 tablespoons white granulated
sugar
2 teaspoons cinnamon

In a small mixing bowl, make revised Popover batter and pour into greased muffin pans. Fill each tin one-quarter full. Mix cinnamon with sugars and sprinkle over batter. Pour more batter into tins until they are half full. Again sprinkle with cinnamon and sugar mixture. Bake in a preheated 400° oven for 20 minutes.

For a glaze, mix a little powdered sugar and milk or milk substitute together and spoon over baked muffins.

Makes 10 muffins

DATE MUFFINS

(*milkless, glutenless, cornless*)

⅓ cup soy flour
½ cup sifted rice flour
½ teaspoon baking powder
1 tablespoon sugar
1 beaten egg (or substitute, see
Appendix A)
1 tablespoon safflower oil

¼ cup milk substitute, or water (see
Appendix A)
2 tablespoons chopped dates
½ cup chopped almonds

Mix dry ingredients together. Combine egg, sugar, and milk substitute (or water), then slowly add to dry ingredients, mixing well. Add dates and almonds to mixture, pour into greased cupcake tins, and bake 25 minutes at 400° or until lightly brown.

Makes 8 muffins

MAIZE MUFFINS

T *(testing for corn—milkless, eggless, glutenless)*

1⅓ cups cornmeal
⅔ cup potato starch
⅔ cup soy flour
½ cup sugar
1 teaspoon salt
4 teaspoons baking powder
1 cube (8 ounces) milkless
  margarine

2 teaspoons baking powder
  mixed with 4 tablespoons safflower oil and 4 tablespoons
  water
1⅓ cups hot soy milk

Preheat oven to 400°. Sift cornmeal, potato starch, and soy flour twice. Combine with other dry ingredients and mix well. Cut in margarine until well blended, and flour looks beaded. In a separate small mixing bowl, combine oil, water, and baking powder, and add to flour mixture. Add hot soy milk. Combine ingredients well, and pour batter into greased muffin tins. Bake for 20 minutes or until golden brown.

Makes 20 muffins

POTATO FLOUR MUFFINS

(milkless, glutenless, cornless)

4 eggs, separated (room
  temperature)
⅛ teaspoon salt
4 teaspoons sugar
½ cup potato flour

1 tablespoon tapioca flour
1 tablespoon baking powder
2 tablespoons ice water

Beat egg whites until stiff but not dry. Beat egg yolks, add salt and sugar, fold into whites. Sift flours and baking powder twice and beat thoroughly into eggs. Stir in ice water. Bake in greased muffin pans at 400° for 15–20 minutes.

Makes 8 muffins

CHEESE-POTATO SCONES

(*glutenless, cornless*)

¾ cup rice flour
⅓ cup mashed potatoes
1 egg (or substitute, see Appendix A)
2 tablespoons margarine

¼ cup milk (or substitute, see Appendix A)
½ teaspoon cream of tartar
1 tablespoon baking powder
½ teaspoon salt
½ cup grated cheese

Mix dry ingredients together with mashed potatoes. Add milk, margarine, beaten egg, and cheese. Roll into balls and place on a greased cookie sheet. Bake 15 minutes at 400°.

Makes 8 scones

RICE BRAN MUFFINS

(*milkless, glutenless, cornless*)

2 tablespoons milkless margarine
¼ cup blackstrap molasses
1 egg (or substitute, see Appendix A)

1 cup rice bran
¾ cup milk substitute (see Appendix A)
3 tablespoons potato flour

Cream margarine, and stir in molasses. Add egg, rice bran, and milk substitute. Let stand until most of the moisture is absorbed. Sift potato flour twice. Stir into bran mixture only until flour is moistened. Fill a greased muffin pan two-thirds full. Bake at 400° for 30 minutes.

Makes 8 muffins

ROQUEFORT BISCUITS

(*eggless, glutenless, cornless*)

½ cup potato starch
½ cup soy flour
¼ teaspoon salt
2 tablespoons baking powder
1 tablespoon sugar
3 tablespoons margarine

⅓ cup milk
¼ cup crumbled Roquefort cheese
3 teaspoons baking powder mixed with 2 tablespoons safflower oil and 2 tablespoons water

Sift flours, salt, baking powder, and sugar twice. With a pastry blender, cut margarine into flour mixture until it resembles small peas. Add milk and cheese, and stir with a fork until dough forms. Add baking powder mixture, and mix well.

Drop biscuits on an ungreased cookie sheet. Bake in preheated 400° oven for 14 minutes or until lightly brown.

Makes 8 biscuits

SWEET POTATO BISCUITS

(*milkless, eggless, cornless*)

1 cup mashed sweet potatoes	1¼ cup flour, sifted
1 cup milk substitute (see Appendix A)	4 teaspoons baking powder
	⅓ cup brown sugar
4 tablespoons milkless margarine, melted	1 tablespoon sugar
	½ teaspoon salt

Mix together sweet potatoes, milk substitute, and margarine, then add sifted flour, baking powder, sugars, and salt. Mix to make a soft dough. Fill a greased muffin pan, and bake at 450° for 15 minutes.

Makes 10 biscuits

APPLE NUT COFFEE CAKE

E (*milkless, eggless, glutenless, cornless*)

Filling:
2 apples, peeled, cored, and chopped
1 tablespoon milkless margarine, melted
1 teaspoon cinnamon (not be used during the elimination diet)
½ cup brown sugar
1 cup sliced almonds

Batter:
1 tablespoon rice flour
1 cup rice flour
1 tablespoon soy flour
½ teaspoon salt
2 teaspoons baking powder
¼ cup sugar
¼ cup milkless margarine
¼ cup milk substitute (see Appendix A)
2 egg substitutes (see Appendix A)

[*167*]

Mix together all ingredients for filling in a small bowl, and set aside.

Sift dry ingredients together. Melt margarine and slowly add sugar. Next add eggs (or substitute) and mix in milk substitute. Add dry ingredients slowly, stirring well. Pour one-third of cake mixture into an 8 × 8 × 2-inch greased pan or small casserole dish, then put one-third filling on top. Layer the rest of the batter and filling according to this procedure. Bake for 30–35 minutes at 375°.

Serves 4

RICEOLA CEREAL

E (*milkless, eggless, glutenless, cornless*)

2 cups puffed brown rice	¼ cup sesame seeds
2 cups puffed millet	¼ cup brown sugar
½ cup sliced almonds	¼ cup raisins

Mix all ingredients together, and serve with milk or a milk substitute. Sweeten with honey.

Variations: add dried dates or dried apples.

Serves 6

CAKES, PIES, AND DESSERTS

In the following recipes, be sure to use a cereal-free, egg-free baking powder when baking powder is called for.

APPLE CRISP

T (*testing for gluten—milkless, eggless, cornless*)

4 apples, cored, peeled, and sliced
2 tablespoons milkless margarine
1 teaspoon cinnamon
½ cup brown sugar
1 cup oats (uncooked)
1 tablespoon soy or arrowroot flour

Place sliced apples in a greased 8 × 2-inch pan. Sprinkle with lemon juice. Mix the rest of the ingredients in a small mixing bowl and sprinkle over apples. Bake at 350° for 20 minutes or until just golden brown.

Variations: Use peaches or cherries (increase brown sugar to ¾ cup)

Serves 6

ALMOND TORTE

(*milkless, glutenless, cornless*)

8 eggs, separated (room temperature)
1¼ cups sugar
Pinch salt
Grated rind of 1 lemon
2¼ cups almonds, blanched and grated
¼ cup rice bread* crumbs

Beat egg yolks with sugar and salt; add grated lemon rind and fold into stiffly beaten egg whites. Add almonds and rice bread crumbs. Bake in a greased and floured 9-inch springform pan at 350° for 45 minutes to 1 hour. Serve with Rum Sauce*.

Serves 6–8

BASIC HONEY CAKE

(glutenless, cornless)

1⅓ cups rice flour
2½ teaspoons baking powder
1 teaspoon salt
½ cup honey
¾ cup milk (or substitute, see
  Appendix A)

½ cup margarine, melted
2 eggs (or substitute, see
  Appendix A)
1 teaspoon vanilla

Sift dry ingredients together and set aside. Mix melted margarine and honey together. Add eggs and vanilla. Add dry ingredients and milk alternately until well blended. Pour into 2 nine-inch cake tins. Bake at 350° for 30–45 minutes.

Serves 8

BLUEBERRY UPSIDE DOWN CAKE

(milkless, glutenless, cornless)

3 tablespoons milkless margarine
1 teaspoon cinnamon
½ cup brown sugar
2 cups frozen blueberries, drained
  with liquid reserved
⅔ cup rice flour
1 tablespoon potato flour
½ teaspoon salt
6 tablespoons sugar
2 tablespoons baking powder

1 egg
1 teaspoon vanilla
½ cup milk substitute (see
  Appendix A)
¼ cup safflower oil

In an 8 × 8 × 2-inch baking pan, melt margarine in a preheated 350° oven. Remove pan from oven, and sprinkle brown sugar and cinnamon over margarine. Top with blueberries and set aside. Sift dry ingredients together twice and pour into a mixing bowl. Add egg, vanilla, milk, and oil. Mix well. Pour mixture over blueberries in baking dish. Bake at 350° for 30 minutes or until golden brown. Allow to cool 10 minutes. Invert on a serving plate. Serve warm or cold.

Serves 6

CAROB CAKE

(glutenless, cornless)

4 eggs, separated (room
  temperature)
1 cup sugar
4 ounces carob chips
½ cup potato starch
1 teaspoon baking powder

Beat egg whites until stiff but not dry. Fold in ½ cup of sugar. Beat egg yolks with ½ cup sugar. Melt carob chips over low heat and blend in with egg yolks and sugar. Add potato starch and baking powder. Mix in a quarter of the egg whites. Fold in remaining egg whites. Pour into 2 greased and floured 8- or 9-inch cake pans. Bake at 350° for 20 minutes. Let cool and remove from pan.

NOTE: Carob chips contain milk by-products.

Serves 8

CARROT NUT CAKE

T *(testing for eggs—milkless, glutenless, cornless)*

2 cups rice flour
2 tablespoons potato flour
1 tablespoon baking powder
1 teaspoon cinnamon
1 teaspoon baking soda
1 teaspoon salt
1 cup oil (safflower, sesame seed)
4 eggs

1 cup honey
1 pound carrots, shredded
½ cup raisins
1 cup almonds, chopped

Mix dry ingredients together and set aside. In a mixing bowl, combine oil, eggs, honey, and shredded carrots. Add carrot mixture slowly to dry ingredients until well blended. Stir in nuts and raisins. Pour into a greased loaf pan and bake at 375° for 1 hour and 15 minutes.

NOTE: With a food processor, carrot shredding is faster.

Serves 8

CHOCOLATE ALMOND TORTE

T (*testing for chocolate—milkless, glutenless, cornless*)

2 cups almonds
¼ cup grated unsweetened
   chocolate
9 eggs, separated (room
   temperature)

1 cup sugar
½ cup fine rice bread* crumbs
   Non-dairy whipped topping
   (cornless)

Chop nuts and set aside ¼ cup for topping. Mix nuts with chocolate. In a separate medium-size bowl, beat egg yolks until light. Then add sugar and beat until creamy. Add nuts, chocolate, and bread crumbs to the egg mixture and mix well. Beat egg whites until stiff but not dry. Mix a quarter of the egg whites into almond mixture. Add another quarter and again mix well. Now gently fold remaining egg whites into mixture. Bake at 350° for 45 minutes in a greased and floured springform pan. Top with whipped topping and remaining nuts.

Serves 8

EGGLESS CHOCOLATE CAKE

(*eggless, cornless*)

1½ cups all-purpose flour
1¼ cups sugar
  3 tablespoons cocoa powder
  2 teaspoons baking powder
  1 teaspoon baking soda
  ¼ teaspoon salt
  1 cup buttermilk

4 tablespoons margarine
1 teaspoon vanilla

Cream together sugar, margarine, and vanilla. Sift together flour, cocoa, baking powder, baking soda, and salt. Add dry ingredients to sugar mixture alternately with buttermilk. Pour into an 8 × 8 × 2-inch greased pan. Bake at 350° for 30 minutes.

Serves 4

GINGERBREAD

(milkless, glutenless, cornless)

1½ cups rice flour
2 tablespoons potato flour
1 tablespoon rice bran
1 teaspoon salt
1½ teaspoons baking soda
1 teaspoon cinnamon
1½ teaspoons ginger
½ cup milkless margarine

1 egg, beaten (or substitute, see Appendix A)
½ cup sugar
1 cup molasses
½–¾ cup very hot water

Sift together flours, rice bran, salt, soda, cinnamon, and ginger. Cream together shortening, sugar, and egg. Beat well. Then add molasses. Alternately add dry mixture and hot water to creamed mixture. First add one-third flour mixture, then one-third water, more flour, then more water and so on until everything is smoothly mixed. Pour into greased and floured 8 × 8× 2-inch pan and bake at 350° for 35–40 minutes.

Serves 8

MAPLE SYRUP CAKE

T *(testing for eggs—milkless, glutenless, cornless)*

1 egg, separated (room temperature)
1 cup brown sugar
1½ teaspoons maple syrup
1 cup non-dairy creamer (cornless variety, see Appendix A under *Milk*)
1⅓ cups rice flour

1 tablespoon potato flour
2 teaspoons baking soda
1 teaspoon salt
1 teaspoon maple flavoring

In a large mixing bowl, beat egg yolk with fork. Add brown sugar and maple syrup and mix well. Add non-dairy creamer. In a separate mixing bowl, blend rice flour, potato flour, soda, and salt, and add to maple syrup mixture. In another mixing bowl, beat egg white until stiff but not dry. Add maple flavoring, and fold into flour mixture. Bake in greased 8 × 8 × 2-inch pan at 350° for 45 minutes.

Serves 8

SWEDISH APPLE TART

(*milkless, eggless, glutenless, cornless*)

6 apples
4 tablespoons brown sugar
1 teaspoon lemon juice
½ cup soy flour
½ cup potato starch

2 tablespoons sugar
1 cube (8 ounces) milkless
margarine

Peel apples and cut into thin slices. Layer slices in a greased ovenproof dish, sprinkling each layer with brown sugar and lemon juice. Sift flour and starch twice. Mix together flours, sugar and margarine, and spread over apple mixture. Bake in 8 × 8 × 2-inch greased pan at 425° for 25 minutes. Top with Vanilla Sauce.*

Serves 6

NEL'S SWEDISH SPONGE CAKE

(*milkless, glutenless,*)

4 eggs, separated (room
temperature)
1 cup sugar
½ cup potato starch
1 teaspoon baking powder
8 ounces non-dairy whipped
topping
¼ cup chopped almonds

Beat the egg whites until stiff but not dry, then fold in ½ cup of sugar. Beat egg yolks and remaining sugar together. Mix yolk mixture and beaten egg whites together gently. Add potato starch and baking powder. Pour into 2 greased and floured 8- or 9-inch layer cake pans. Bake at 350° for 20 minutes. Let cool and remove from pan. Fill and top with non-dairy topping. Sprinkle with nuts.

This is a delicious heirloom recipe.

Serves 8

WAR CAKE

T (*testing for gluten—milkless, eggless, cornless*)

1 cup brown sugar
1 cup water
⅓ cup safflower oil
1 cup raisins
1 teaspoon cinnamon
1 teaspoon ground cloves
½ teaspoon nutmeg
2 cups flour
½ teaspoon baking powder
½ teaspoon salt
½ teaspoon baking soda

Boil together brown sugar, water, oil, raisins, cinnamon, cloves, and nutmeg for 3 minutes. Cool thoroughly. Add flour sifted with baking powder, salt, and soda. Mix well. Pour into a greased bundt pan, and bake 45 minutes at 350°.

Serves 6–8

BASIC RICE PIE CRUST

E (*milkless, eggless, glutenless, cornless*)

1 cup rice flour
¼ teaspoon salt
2 tablespoons soy flour
6 tablespoons milkless margarine
4 tablespoons ice water

Measure flours and salt into a mixing bowl. Cut in margarine until flour looks beaded. Sprinkle in ice water one tablespoon at a time until flour is completely moistened. Shape dough into a ball, flatten into a round, and place between two strips of waxed paper. Roll pastry 2 inches larger than size of intended pie pan. Peel off top paper, place pastry paper side up in pan, peel off paper, and ease pastry into pan. Bake as directed.

Double the recipe for a 2-crust pie.

CEREAL PIE CRUST

(milkless, eggless, glutenless)

1½ cups crushed cereal (Corn
    Bran, Rice Crispies, Rice Chex)
4 tablespoons milkless
    margarine, melted
¼ cup brown sugar

Grease a 9-inch pie pan or springform pan. In a mixing bowl, combine crushed cereal, margarine, and sugar. Press onto bottom and sides of prepared pie pan. Bake 8–10 minutes in a preheated 375° oven. Cool.

ALMOND CEREAL CRUST

(milkless, eggless, glutenless)

1 cup crushed cereal (wheat-free)
⅓ cup ground almonds
4 tablespoons milkless margarine,
    melted
⅓ cup brown sugar

Grease a 9-inch pie pan or springform pan. In a mixing bowl, combine crushed cereal, almonds, margarine, and sugar. Press onto bottom and sides of prepared pie pan. Bake 8–10 minutes in preheated 375° oven. Cool.

ALMOND PIE CRUST

E *(milkless, eggless, glutenless, cornless)*

1½ cups finely ground almonds   2 tablespoons milkless margarine
2 tablespoons sugar

Grease a 9-inch pie pan. Combine ingredients and press into bottom and sides of prepared pie pan. Place in a preheated 375° oven. Bake 10 minutes. Cool.

KASSARI CHEESE PIE CRUST

E (*milkless, eggless, glutenless, cornless*)

1¼ cups rice flour
½ cup finely grated Kassari cheese
  (imported/sheep)
¼ teaspoon salt
⅓ cup safflower oil
2 tablespoons ice water

In a mixing bowl, combine flour, cheese, and salt. Add oil, and mix until dough is the size of small peas. Sprinkle in water one tablespoon at a time until all the flour is moistened. Shape dough into a ball, flatten into a round, and place between two strips of waxed paper. Roll pastry 2 inches larger than size of intended pie pan. Peel off top paper, place pastry paper side up in pan, peel off paper, and ease pastry into pan. Bake as directed.
  Double the recipe for a 2-crust pie.

PUMPKIN TOFU PIE

(*milkless, glutenless, cornless*)

2 eggs
1 cup mashed tofu
1 sixteen-ounce can pumpkin
¾ cup dark brown sugar
½ teaspoon salt
1½ teaspoons pumpkin pie spice
1 teaspoon vanilla
⅔ cup soy milk
1 9-inch unbaked Basic Rice Pie
  Crust*

Preheat oven to 375°. Beat eggs in a large bowl. Add tofu and beat until creamy. Stir in remaining ingredients until well blended. Pour into a prepared pastry shell. Bake for 45 minutes.

Serves 8

PUMPKIN PIE

E (*milkless, eggless, glutenless, cornless*)

¾ cup brown sugar
1 cup canned pumpkin
2 tablespoons tapioca flour
1 tablespoon pumpkin pie spice
2 cups milk substitute (see
  Appendix A)
1 9-inch baked Basic Rice
  Pie Crust*

Mix sugar, pumpkin, tapioca, spice, and milk substitute in a medium-size mixing bowl. Pour into pie shell and bake for 15 minutes at 425°.

Serves 8

BLUEBERRY PIE I

(milkless, eggless, glutenless, cornless)

Pastry for a 2-crust pie
(Almond* or Basic Rice*)
1 ten-ounce package frozen
blueberries
1 tablespoon soy flour

½ cup sugar
1 tablespoon milkless margarine
1 tablespoon lemon juice

Prepare pastry and roll out to fit an 8-inch pie pan. Combine blueberries, flour, and sugar. Stir in lemon juice and pour into pastry shell. Top with second crust. Make slits in crust, and bake in preheated 400° oven for 45 minutes or until crust is golden.

Serves 8

BLUEBERRY PIE II

(milkless, eggless, glutenless)

Pastry for a 2-crust pie*
1 quart fresh blueberries
½ cup sugar
1 cup water
1 teaspoon cornstarch

1 teaspoon oil
1 teaspoon lemon juice
½ teaspoon vanilla

Prepare pastry and roll out to fit an 8-inch pie pan. In a large saucepan, dissolve sugar in water. Add blueberries and cook until they are tender. Combine cornstarch, oil, and lemon juice in a separate bowl, add to blueberries, and cook until thickened. Remove from heat and add vanilla. Pour into pastry shell. Top with second crust, and bake at 400° for 45 minutes or until crust is golden.

Serves 8

CRANBERRY PIE

(milkless, glutenless,cornless)

2 cups sugar
1 cup water
1 pound fresh cranberries
2 tablespoons tapioca flour

¼ teaspoon salt
3 tablespoons milkless margarine
2 egg yolks, beaten
1 9-inch unbaked Basic Rice
Pie Crust*

In a large saucepan, dissolve ¾ cup of sugar in water. Add cranberries and cook until they stop popping. Combine tapioca, remaining sugar, salt, margarine, and egg yolks. Add a small amount of cooked cranberries to tapioca mixture. Mix well. Then add mixture to remaining cranberries and cook until thickened. When mixture is thick and clear, pour into pastry shell. Bake in a preheated 400° oven until crust is golden.

Serves 8

CAROB MOUSSE I

(glutenless, cornless)

4 eggs (room temperature)
4 ounces carob chips
4 tablespoons margarine
2 tablespoons sugar

Separate egg yolks and egg whites into 2 separate bowls (glass or metal—never rubber). In a saucepan, melt carob chips and margarine together over low heat. Remove pan from heat and whisk until carob mixture thickens slightly. Pour into the mixing bowl with egg yolks and whisk one more minute. In a separate bowl, beat egg whites until stiff but not dry. Gently stir in sugar. Now add half of the beaten egg whites to carob mixture. Stir carefully, blending all the ingredients together. Using a rubber spatula, fold in remaining egg whites. The correct motion is to start with the spatula in the middle of the bowl and fold upward in a circular motion. Fold until mixture is thoroughly blended. Pour into a serving bowl and refrigerate for at least 3 hours.

NOTE: Carob chips have milk by-products in them.

Serves 4

CAROB MOUSSE II

T (*testing for milk—eggless, glutenless, cornless*)

1 envelope unflavored gelatin
¼ cup cold water
4 ounces carob chips

10 ounces heavy cream
¼ cup sugar
1 teaspoon pure vanilla extract

Soften gelatin in cold water, then dissolve it over hot water. Cool to luke-warm. In a saucepan, melt carob chips over low heat. Allow to cool slightly. Combine carob chips, sugar, heavy cream, and vanilla. Gradually add gelatin, beating well after each addition. Continue beating until thick. Pour into a serving bowl and chill for up to 3–4 hours.

Serves 4

DESSERT FROSTINGS AND SAUCES

ALMOND PASTE

(*milkless, glutenless, cornless*)

¾ pound ground almonds
1 cup sugar

1 tablespoon lemon juice
4 egg whites (room temperature)

Add ground almonds to sugar and lemon juice. Mix well. Beat egg whites until stiff but not dry. Mix a quarter of the egg whites into almond mixture, then gently fold remaining egg whites into mixture.

Makes 1 cup

CAROB SYRUP I

T (*testing for corn—milkless, eggless, glutenless*)

1 cup sugar
½ cup carob powder
½ cup light corn syrup

½ cup water
½ teaspoon vanilla

Combine sugar and carob in a saucepan. Blend in corn syrup and water. Stir in a figure eight motion to dissolve sugar. Simmer gently for 8 minutes, stirring occasionally. Add vanilla extract, and remove saucepan from heat. Cool, then store in refrigerator.

Makes 1 cup

CAROB SYRUP II

E (*milkless, eggless, glutenless, cornless*)

½ cup carob powder
4 tablespoons tapioca flour
½ teaspoon salt
1 cup sugar

½ cup brown sugar
1 cup water
1 teaspoon vanilla

Combine powder, tapioca flour, salt, and sugar. Gradually add water, bringing to a boil. Boil gently for 5 minutes, stirring frequently. Remove from heat, add vanilla, and store in refrigerator.

Makes 1 cup

MAPLE SYRUP

E (*milkless, eggless, glutenless, cornless*)

3 cups sugar
½ cup brown sugar
2 tablespoons milkless margarine

2 cups water
1 teaspoon vanilla
1 teaspoon maple extract

Heat water, add margarine, dissolve sugar, bring mixture to a boil, and boil gently for 7 minutes. Remove from heat. Cool slightly. Add vanilla and maple extract.

Makes 2 cups

BASIC FROSTING

(*milkless, eggless, glutenless, cornless*)

¼ cup soy baby formula (cornless)
1 pound confectioners sugar
1 teaspoon vanilla
⅔ cup Crisco

Beat all ingredients with an electric mixer until smooth and creamy.

CREAM CHEESE FROSTING

T (*testing for milk—eggless, glutenless, cornless*)

¼ cup evaporated milk
¾ of a 1-pound box confectioners
    sugar

1 teaspoon vanilla
¼ cup cream cheese
½ cup Crisco

Beat all ingredients with an electric mixer until smooth and creamy.

Variations: May add extract other than vanilla: maple, rum, almond, etc.

RUM SAUCE I

(*milkless, glutenless*)

2 eggs, separated (room
    temperature)

⅓ cup sugar
1 teaspoon rum extract

Beat egg yolks and sugar until thick. Add rum extract and fold mixture into stiffly beaten egg whites.

Makes ½ cup

VANILLA SAUCE

E (*milkless, eggless, glutenless, cornless*)

2 tablespoons milkless margarine
2 tablespoons arrowroot flour
1 cup boiling water

2 tablespoons sugar
1 teaspoon vanilla

Melt margarine, add flour, and stir until it bubbles. Add boiling water and sugar. Stirring constantly with a wooden spoon but not allowing the spoon to surface, cook until smooth. Remove from heat and stir in vanilla.

Makes 1⅓ cups

RUM SAUCE II

(*milkless, glutenless*)

Follow instructions for Vanilla Sauce* but add rum extract instead of vanilla at the end.

Makes 1⅓ cups

COOKIES, TREATS, AND CANDIES

In the following recipes, be sure to use a cereal-free, egg-free baking powder when baking powder is called for.

BROWN RICE BROWNIES

T (*testing for chocolate—milkless, glutenless, cornless*)

2 ounces semi-sweet chocolate
⅓ cup milkless margarine
⅔ cup brown rice flour
1 tablespoon potato flour
½ teaspoon salt
1½ teaspoons baking powder
1 cup sugar
2 eggs, well beaten
 Chopped nuts (optional)

Melt chocolate and margarine in a microwave or over a double boiler. Remove from heat and stir in sugar and eggs. Beat until creamy. Sift flours, salt, and baking powder together twice, and add to chocolate mixture slowly. Pour into a greased 8 × 8 × 2-inch pan and bake at 350° for 30–35 minutes.

NOTE: These brownies taste a little like brownies made with whole-wheat flour.

Serves 8

When using rice flour for cookies, it is helpful to refrigerate the cookie mixture for at least an hour prior to cooking.

CAROB CHIP COOKIES

(glutenless, cornless)

½ cup honey
⅓ cup brown sugar
½ cup margarine, melted
1 egg (or substitute, see Appendix A)
1 teaspoon vanilla

2 teaspoons baking powder
½ teaspoon salt
1 cup rice flour
½ cup soya flour
2 tablespoons potato flour
12 ounces carob chips

Sift dry ingredients together. Cream honey and margarine and add egg and vanilla. Slowly add dry ingredients, and then carob chips. Drop by teaspoonfuls on a greased baking sheet. Bake at 400° for 10–12 minutes.

Makes 2 dozen

CAROB PEANUT BUTTER FUDGE BARS

(eggless, glutenless, cornless)

4 tablespoons margarine
3 cups carob chips

2 cups peanut butter
6 cups Rice Crispies cereal

In a saucepan over very low heat, melt together margarine, carob chips, and peanut butter. Remove from heat and stir in cereal. Spread in 9 × 13-inch greased pan. Chill for 30 minutes and then cut into bars.

Makes 2 dozen

BANANA-NUT OATMEAL COOKIES

T *(testing for gluten—milkless, eggless, cornless)*

3 ripe bananas, mashed
⅓ cup safflower oil
2 cups quick-cooking rolled oats

1 cup chopped almonds
1 teaspoon vanilla
½ teaspoon salt

In a large mixing bowl mash bananas, add other ingredients, and mix well. Drop by rounded tablespoonfuls on an ungreased cookie sheet. Bake at 350° for 20–25 minutes.

Makes 3½ dozen

CHERRY BARS

E (*milkless, eggless, glutenless, cornless*)

6 tablespoons milkless margarine
½ cup brown sugar
1 tablespoon rice bran
2 tablespoons potato flour
⅞ cup rice flour
2 envelopes unflavored gelatin

1 teaspoon almond extract
½ cup chopped cherries
½ cup cold water
1½ cups sugar
½ cup warm water
½ cup chopped almonds

Cream margarine and brown sugar together. Sift flours and bran twice. Add flours to margarine and sugar, and mix well. Spread in a greased 9 × 13-inch pan and bake at 350° for 25 minutes. Cool. Meanwhile in a separate bowl, dissolve gelatin in cold water. Set aside. Boil sugar and warm water for 2 minutes, then combine with gelatin mixture, and beat until stiff. Add almond extract, cherries, and almonds, and pour on top of baked mixture. Let set and cut into squares.

Serves 8

CHOCOLATE SPRITZ COOKIES

(*milkless, glutenless, cornless*)

½ cup shortening
2 tablespoons milkless margarine
½ cup sugar
1 egg
½ teaspoon vanilla
½ teaspoon almond extract

2 tablespoons cocoa
1 cup rice flour
2 tablespoons potato flour
¼ teaspoon baking powder
¼ teaspoon salt

Cream together shortening and margarine until fluffy. Add sugar and beat until creamy. Add egg, vanilla, and almond extract, and beat well. Add cocoa. Sift flours, baking powder, and salt together twice. Add to shortening mixture; dough will be stiff. Shape into 2 rolls, wrap in wax paper, and refrigerate for at least 1 hour. Fill a cookie press with a quarter of the dough at a time. Form desired shapes on an ungreased baking sheet. Bake at 375° 8–10 minutes.

Makes 2½ dozen

MERINGUE COOKIES

(milkless, glutenless, cornless)

2 egg whites (room temperature)   ¾ cup sugar
½ teaspoon cream of tartar   Nuts (almonds, carob chips, etc.)

Beat egg whites until stiff but not dry. Add cream of tartar. Slowly beat in sugar, then add nuts or chips. Drop mixture onto a cookie sheet lined with wax paper. Heat oven at 350° for 30 minutes. Put cookies into oven, and turn off heat. Do not open oven or remove cookies until the next morning.

Makes 1½ dozen

OATMEAL LACE COOKIES

(milkless, eggless, cornless)

½ cup milkless margarine, melted   1 teaspoon salt
1¼ cups brown sugar   2 teaspoons baking powder
½ teaspoon vanilla   ¼ cup water
¼ cup rice flour   2 cups quick-cooking rolled oats
½ cup soy flour   ½ cup slivered almonds

Beat together melted margarine, brown sugar, and vanilla until creamy. Mix flours, salt, and baking powder, and sift. Add flour mixture alternately with water to sugar mixture. Stir in rolled oats and nuts. Chill for 2 hours. Preheat oven to 350°. Drop by teaspoon on a greased baking sheet about 2 inches apart. Bake until lightly brown for about 12–15 minutes.

Makes 2 dozen

ORANGE CORNMEAL COOKIES

T *(testing for citrus—milkless, glutenless)*

¾ cup brown sugar   1 cup cornmeal
⅓ cup honey   ¼ cup soy flour
1 egg   2 tablespoons potato flour
⅓ cup milkless margarine   2 tablespoons grated orange rind
1 teaspoon vanilla   ⅓ cup orange juice

Blend together brown sugar, honey, vanilla, and margarine. Add eggs and beat well. Mix in orange juice and orange rind. Slowly add flour mixture. Drop cookies on a greased cookie sheet. Bake at 375° for 12–15 minutes.

Serves 8

SOFT MOLASSES COOKIES

T (*testing for gluten—milkless, eggless, cornless*)

1 cup blackstrap molasses
1 teaspoon cream of tartar
1 cup sugar
3 tablespoons safflower oil
3 tablespoons water
2 teaspoons baking powder
(egg-free)

1½ cups milkless margarine
2 teaspoons baking soda
4 cups flour
1 cup water
1 teaspoon ginger
1 teaspoon salt

Mix together molasses, tartar, and sugar. In a separate bowl, beat together oil, water, and baking powder. Add this mixture to molasses mixture. Stir in baking soda, flour, water, ginger, and salt. Chill mixture for 2 hours. Drop on a cookie sheet from a spoon, and bake at 375° for 8–12 minutes.

Makes 5 dozen

RAISIN COOKIES

(*milkless, eggless, cornless*)

1 cup brown sugar
2 tablespoons milkless margarine
1 cup raisins
1 cup water

½ teaspoon salt
1 teaspoon cinnamon
1½ cups flour
½ teaspoon ginger

Cook together sugar, margarine, raisins, water and salt. Cool completely. Sift dry ingredients together and stir into cooled mixture. Drop by teaspoonfuls onto a baking sheet, and bake at 350° for 15 minutes.

Makes approximately 3 dozen

SESAME SEED COOKIES

(milkless, glutenless, cornless)

2 cups rice flour
2 tablespoons soy flour
1 teaspoon baking powder
½ teaspoon salt
1 teaspoon vanilla
2 eggs, beaten (or substitute, see Appendix A)

¼ cup safflower oil
¾ cup honey
¼ cup molasses
1 cup sesame seeds
¼ cup chopped dates

Sift together dry ingredients and set aside. Combine oil, honey, molasses, eggs, and vanilla, then add dry mix slowly. Stir in sesame seeds. Refrigerate 12 hours to overnight. When ready to bake, form batter into balls, flatten them with a greased end of a glass, press one chopped date in the center of each, and bake on a greased cookie sheet for 8–10 minutes at 375°.

Makes 3 dozen cookies

NATURE'S MACAROONS

T *(testing for eggs—milkless, glutenless, cornless)*

2 egg whites
¼ cup honey
¼ cup molasses
1 teaspoon vanilla

¼ cup rice flour
2½ cups unsweetened coconut
1 teaspoon milkless margarine

Beat egg whites until stiff. Combine molasses, honey, vanilla, and margarine and fold into beaten egg whites. Add rice flour and coconut. Refrigerate. Shape into balls. Flatten to rectangular cookies on a greased baking sheet, and bake 10–15 minutes at 325°. Store in refrigerator.

Makes 2 dozen

ALMOND SESAME CANDY I

E *(milkless, eggless, glutenless, cornless)*

1 cup brown sugar
½ cup water
½ cup honey

½ pound sesame seeds
½ pound chopped blanched almonds

Mix sugar and honey in a saucepan, add water slowly, and cook over low heat until mixture forms soft balls. Remove from heat. Let cool slightly. Add almond and sesame seeds. Pour into 8 × 8 × 2-inch greased pan. Allow to cool. Cut into squares.

Makes 16 squares

ALMOND SESAME CANDY II

E (*milkless, eggless, glutenless, cornless*)

¾ cup honey
¼ cup sugar
½ cup brown sugar

1 cup blanched almonds
1 cup sesame seeds
½ teaspoon vanilla

In a saucepan, bring honey and sugar to boiling, stirring constantly to dissolve sugar. Cook until a candy thermometer reads 220°. Reduce heat, add nuts and sesame seeds, and cook 10 minutes more or until nuts and seeds turn golden. Remove from heat, stir in vanilla, and pour candy onto a greased cookie sheet. Cool. Cut into squares.

Makes 12–15 bars

SWEET RICE FLOUR BALLS

E (*milkless, eggless, glutenless, cornless*)

1½ cups sweet rice flour (found in Japanese section of most markets)
⅔ cup coconut milk (see below)

¼ teaspoon salt
¼ cup brown sugar
1 cup unsweetened coconut

Coconut milk: 1 cup unsweetened coconut, ⅔ cup hot water. Mix in a blender until milk forms. Drain through a sieve lined with cheesecloth.

Combine 1¼ cups rice flour, coconut milk, and salt, and mix until a creamy paste forms. Work mixture into balls. Roll balls in remaining ¼ cup of rice flour mixed with brown sugar. Drop into 3 quarts of boiling water. Stir constantly to prevent sticking. Boil 5–7 minutes until balls rise to surface. Allow to drain on paper towel. While balls are still warm, roll in the coconut.

Makes 2 dozen balls

PEANUT BUTTER CRISP

E (*milkless, eggless, glutenless, cornless*)

½ cup packed brown sugar
½ cup peanut butter
¼ cup canned milk substitute
   (baby formula may be used; see
   Appendix A)
2¼ cups Rice Crispies cereal

In a medium saucepan, combine brown sugar, peanut butter, and canned milk substitute. Bring to a simmer, stirring constantly until sugar is dissolved and peanut butter is melted. Remove from heat. Stir in cereal, and drop by the teaspoonful onto waxed paper.

Makes 2 dozen

ALMOND CAROB FUDGE

(*milkless, eggless, glutenless*)

2 cups sugar
¾ cup milk substitute (see
   Appendix A)
¼ cup carob powder

2 tablespoons milkless margarine
1 teaspoon vanilla
¼ cup chopped almonds

In a medium saucepan, combine sugar, milk substitute, carob, and margarine. Bring to a boil, and stir until mixture is smooth. Boil to 240° on a candy thermometer, softball stage. Remove from fire and beat with a wooden spoon until thick and creamy. Stir in vanilla and nuts. Pour into an 8 × 8 × 2-inch greased pan. Cool until hard. Cut into squares.

Makes 16 squares

CAROB BON BONS

(*glutenless, cornless*)

12 ounces carob chips
½ cup confectioners sugar
3 tablespoons margarine

3 egg yolks, beaten
Confectioners sugar

In a saucepan, melt margarine and chips over low heat and combine with sugar. Remove from heat, add beaten egg yolks, and blend well. Transfer to a metal or glass mixing bowl and chill 1–2 hours. Shape into 1-inch balls, then roll them in confectioners sugar. Store in refrigerator.

Makes 2½ dozen

CAROB CLUSTER

(*eggless, glutenless, cornless*)

½ pound carob chips   2 tablespoons water
1 cup rice puff cereal   ¼ cup brown sugar
¼ cup honey   ¼ cup margarine

Melt carob chips in top of a double boiler. Add melted carob to sugar, honey, and margarine. Heat continuously; add water. When mixture is hot enough to form a soft ball, remove from heat. Cool slightly. Pour over rice puffs on a greased cookie sheet or waxed paper. Cool. Break off into separate pieces.

Makes 2 dozen pieces

NOUGAT

(*milkless, glutenless, cornless*)

1 pound almonds, blanched   2 tablespoons Almond Paste*
1¼ cups sugar   2 tablespoons honey
½ cup honey   ¼ cup rice flour
2 tablespoons milk substitute
   (see Appendix A)

Toast almonds in a moderate oven (350°) until golden brown. Place them in a saucepan, add sugar and honey, and melt over low heat. Add milk substitute, almond paste, and 2 tablespoons honey. Remove from heat and beat with a wooden spoon until mixture becomes smooth. Sprinkle rice flour over wax paper, pour mixture on it, and cool. Cut into squares.

Makes 1½ dozen

ITALIAN ICES

E (*milkless, eggless, glutenless, cornless*)

1 cup sugar
1 cup water
3 cups fresh peaches, or canned
  peaches (no syrup—must be
  canned in own juice)

In a saucepan, dissolve sugar into water. Boil 1 minute, reduce heat, and stir until it becomes syruplike.

In a blender or food processor, purée peaches until smooth. Add cooled syrup mixture and mix together. Pour peach and syrup mixture into flexible ice cube containers and freeze until solid. Once frozen, put cubes into a blender or food processor and "chop" until just snowlike. Serve immediately.

Variations: Banana ices
           Champagne ices—increase sugar to 2 cups

Serves 8–10

BEVERAGES

APPLE-BANANA DRINK

E (*milkless, eggless, glutenless, cornless*)

2 bananas, mashed
1 apple, cored, peeled, and chopped

2 cups apple juice
¼ cup honey

Place all ingredients in a blender and blend until smooth. Chill and serve.

Makes 2¼ cups

COOL BANANA PICKUP

E (*milkless, eggless, glutenless, cornless*)

2 medium bananas, mashed
2 cups soy milk
⅓ cup honey

Mix together in a blender. Chill.

Makes 2 cups

CAROB-NUT DRINK

E (*milkless, eggless, glutenless, cornless*)

½ cup blanched almonds
3 tablespoons water
3 tablespoons carob powder
2 tablespoons honey
2 cups milk substitute (see
   Appendix A)

Place nuts in a blender with water and blend until smooth. Add remaining ingredients and blend until smooth. Refrigerate and serve.

Makes 2¼ cups

MAPLE DELIGHT

E (*milkless, eggless, glutenless, cornless*)

½ cup Maple Syrup*
1½ cups milk substitute (see
   Appendix A)
1 egg substitute (see
   Appendix A)

Mix together in a blender. Chill.

Makes 2 cups

TOFU COCONUT MILK

E (*milkless, eggless, glutenless, cornless*)

2 cups mashed tofu
2 cups grated unsweetened coconut

½ cup honey
2 teaspoons vanilla

Put all ingredients in a blender and blend until smooth. Pour through a sieve lined with cheesecloth. Chill 3 hours.

Makes 2 cups

VEGETABLE COCKTAIL

E (*milkless, eggless, glutenless, cornless*)

1 medium cucumber, peeled and
   grated
½ cup grated carrots
2 cups tomato juice
2 tablespoons chopped scallions
1 teaspoon miso
1 teaspoon salt
2 drops hot pepper sauce
   Dash cayenne pepper
   Chopped parsley

Into a blender, put grated cucumber, carrots, tomato juice, miso, salt, hot pepper, and pepper. Run blender on purée. Strain through a sieve lined with cheesecloth. Chill. Serve with sprinkles of parsley.

Makes 2¼ cups

APPENDIX A

Substitutes (specific products listed here are not necessarily the only ones available —they are just suggestions)

Milk

- Soy Moo Non-Dairy Creamer (cornless)
- Lucerne Frozen Non-Dairy Creamer (contains corn syrup)
- Rich's Rich Whip
- Soyamel (powdered soy milk)
- Mocha Mix
- Coffee Rich
- Jolly Joan Soy Quik

Watch out for ingredients: milk, non-fat milk, milk protein, casein, dried milk solids, whey, and sodium caseinate.

NOTE: Non-dairy creamers usually contain corn syrup, and some milk substitutes can contain corn syrup. Make sure to check the label.

Egg

- Gold Harvest Egg Replacer
- Jolly Joan Egg Replacer
- 1 teaspoon unflavored gelatin + 3 tablespoons cold water + 2 tablespoons and 1 teaspoon boiling water
- 1½ tablespoons oil + 1½ tablespoons water + 1 teaspoon baking powder (cereal-free/egg-free)

Watch out for ingredients: albumin, ovalbumin, egg, egg products.

NOTE: Some commercial brands contain milk by-products.

Wheat

- Rice, potato, soy, tapioca, lima bean, and arrowroot flours and cornmeal
- Ener-G Gluten-Free Mix
- Golden Harvest Rice Mix
- Jolly Joan Rice Mix

- Jolly Joan Pure Rice Bran
- Jolly Joan Pure Rice Polish
- Jolly Joan Brown Rice Baking Mix
- Fearn (Soy/o) Rice Baking Mix
- Cellu Gluten-Free Bread Mix

Watch out for ingredients: flour, wheat, starch, gluten, gliadin, cereal, malt.

Corn

May use same substitutes as for wheat; also may use wheat.
Watch out for ingredients: corn, zein, maize.

Baking Powder

- Featherweight (cereal-free) Baking Powder
- Cellu (cereal-free) Baking Powder

Mayonnaise

- Hains Eggless Mayonnaise
- Featherweight Eggless Mayonnaise

Pasta

- De Boles Spaghetti—100% corn
- De Boles Noodle Ribbons—100% corn
- De Boles Macaroni—100% corn

APPENDIX B

Food Families

Apple—apple, crabapple, pear, quince
Arrowroot—arrowroot
Banana—banana
Berry—blackberry, boysenberry, raspberry
Blueberry (heath)—blueberry, huckleberry, cranberry
Buckwheat—buckwheat, rhubarb, garden sorrel
Caper—caper
Cashew—cashew, pistachio, mango
Chinese Water Chestnut—water chestnut
Citrus—grapefruit, lemon, lime, orange, tangerine
Coffee—coffee
Cola Nut (Stercula)—chocolate, cocoa, cola nut
Composite—globe artichoke, Jerusalem artichoke, chicory, endive, escarole, lettuce, safflower seed, tarragon
Crustacean—crab, lobster, shrimp
Ebony—date plum, persimmon
Elm—slippery elm tea
Fish—all true fish, either freshwater or saltwater, including tuna, sardine, catfish, trout and crappie
Fungi—mushroom, yeast
Ginger—cardamom, turmeric, ginger
Goosefoot—beet, beet sugar, spinach, Swiss chard
Gourd (melon)—canteloupe, cucumber, honeydew, pumpkin, squash, watermelon, zucchini
Grape—raisin
Grass—wheat, corn, rice, oats, barley, rye, wild rice, cane sugar, millet, bamboo shoots
Honey—honey, bee nectar
Honeysuckle—elderberry
Iris—saffron
Laurel—avocado, cinnamon, bay leaves, sassafras
Legume (pea)—kidney bean, lima bean, navy bean, soy bean, carob, green pea, split pea, alfalfa, lentil, green bean
Lily—asparagus, chive, leek, onion, shallot, garlic, sassaparilla
Linden—linden tea
Linseed—flax, flaxseed

Mallow—althea root tea, cottonseed, okra
Maple—maple sugar
Meat Family—beef (veal, milk, butter, cheese, gelatin), pork (bacon, ham), mutton (lamb)
Mint—balm, basil, marjoram, rosemary, sage, thyme, savory, spearmint, mint, peppermint
Mollusc—oyster, clam, abalone, mussel
Morning Glory—sweet potato, yam
Mulberry—breadfruit, fig, mulberry
Mustard—mustard green, cabbage, cauliflower, collard, Chinese cabbage, broccoli, brussel sprout, radish, turnip, watercress, kale
Myrtle—allspice, guava, clove
Nettle—hop, oregano
Nightshade—eggplant, cayenne, bell pepper, red pepper, paprika, tomato, potato, pimento
Nutmeg—mace, nutmeg
Olive—black olive, green olive
Orchid—vanilla
Palm—coconut, dates
Parsley—anise, carrot, celery, caraway seed, parsley, coriander, dill, cumin, fennel
Pepper—black and white pepper
Pineapple—pineapple
Plum—plum, cherry, peach, apricot, nectarine, wild cherry, almond
Rose—blackthorn, strawberry
Seaweed—dulse, kelp
Sesame—sesame seed
Spurge—tapioca
Tea—green tea
Walnut—English walnut, black walnut, pecan, hickory nut, butternut

APPENDIX C

Allergy Organizations and Resources

American Academy of Allergy
611 E. Wells Street
Milwaukee, WI 53202

American Allergy Association
P.O. Box 640
Menlo Park, CA 94025

American Association for Clinical Immunology and Allergy
P.O. Box 912, DTS
Omaha, NE 68101

American Association for the Study of Headache
5252 N. Western Avenue
Chicago, IL 60625

American Board of Allergy and Immunology
University City Science Center
3624 Market Street
Philadelphia, PA 19104

American Broncho-Esophagological
37 Lawrence Avenue
Fairfield, ME 04937

American Celiac Society (gluten sensitivity)
45 Gifford Avenue
Jersey City, NJ 07304

American College of Allergists
2141 14th Street
Boulder, CO 80302

American College of Gastroenterology (digestive)
299 Broadway
New York, NY 10017

American Council of Otolaryngology
1100 17th Street, N.W., Suite 602
Washington, D.C. 20036

American Dermatologic Society of Allergy and Immunology
University of Missouri Medical Center, M173
807 Stadium Road
Columbia, MO 65212

American Dietetic Association
430 N. Michigan Avenue
Chicago, IL 60611

American Digestive Disease Society
420 Lexington Avenue
New York, NY 10017

American Laryngological Association
40 William M. Trible M.P.
Washington Hospital Center
Washington, D.C. 20010

American Laryngological, Rhinological and Otological Association
(ear, nose, throat)
c/o Ann R. Holm
2954 Dorman Road
Broomal, PA 19008

American Lung Association (respiratory diseases)
1740 Broadway
New York, NY 10019

American Rhinologic Society
Penn Park Medical Center
2929 Baltimore, Suite 105
Kansas City, MO 64108

American Society of Ophthalmologic and Otolaryngologic Allergy
c/o William P. King
1415 Third Street, Suite 507
Corpus Christi, TX 78404

Association for the Advancement of Health Education
1201 16th Street, N.W.
Washington, D.C. 20036

Association of Allergist for Mycological Investigations
444 Hermann Professional Building
Houston, TX 77030

Association for the Care of Asthma (formerly the Association of Convalescent
Homes and Hospitals for Asthmatic Children)
Spring Valley Road
Ossining, NY 10562

Asthma and Allergy Foundation of America
801 Second Avenue
New York, NY 10017

Hay Fever Prevention Society
Rosewall Gardens, Suite 2G
2300 Sedgwick Avenue
Bronx, NY 10468

International Correspondence Society of Allergists
139 Grant Avenue
Columbus, OH 43215

National Foundation for Asthma
P.O. Box 50304
Tucson, AZ 85703

National Foundation for Ileitis and Colitis (intestinal inflammation)
295 Madison Avenue
New York, NY 10017

National Migraine Foundation
5214 N. Western Avenue
Chicago, IL 60625

Southwest Allergy Forum
Department of Continuing Education
University of New Mexico School of Medicine
Albuquerque, NM 87131

APPENDIX D

Allergy Medical Care Centers

Robert B. Brigham, Boston, Massachusetts

Duke University Medical Center, Division of Allergy and Respiratory Disease, Durham, North Carolina

Mayo Clinic Allergy Unit, Rochester, Minnesota

National Jewish Hospital and Research Center, Denver, Colorado

Roosevelt Hospital, R.A. Cooke Institute of Allergy, New York, New York

University of Wisconsin Clinical Science Center, Allergy Division, Madison, Wisconsin

INGREDIENT GLOSSARY

BEANS AND LEGUMES

Kidney beans, pinto beans, garbanzo beans (chick peas), and lentils are all prepared by washing, shelling, and boiling for 30 minutes. This is followed by simmering until tender. Although these vegetables are all high in protein, they are still considered incomplete proteins. The exception to this is soybeans, the one legume that is a complete protein. If an allergy to legumes is suspected, then the recipes containing tofu and soybean seasonings must be omitted. Also beware of recipes containing extracts from the vanilla bean.

CHEESES

Cheese as a source of protein is too important to ignore. Therefore cheeses containing no cow's milk need to be included in the allergic individual's diet. The choices are cheeses made from the milk of the ewe (sheep), goat, reindeer, and buffalo. Cheeses made from the milk of the buffalo and reindeer are almost impossible to find. However, cheeses made from ewe's and goat's milk are a little easier to find in their pure state. The safer cheeses are those that are imported. In the United States *most* companies add cow's milk to every cheese. Please check your labels!

The availability of ewe's (sheep) and goat's milk cheese is seasonal. The best season for sheep's milk cheese is the end of autumn to the end of winter (about March). The best season for goat's milk cheese is the end of spring, through summer, to the beginning of autumn.

The following are varieties of sheep's and goat's milk cheeses available:

Cheeses made from ewe's (sheep) milk

Annot. This cheese is made either from sheep or goat's milk. It has a mild nutty flavor and is used in desserts.

Alemtijo. Goat's milk is sometimes added to this cheese.

Feta. A very tangy tasting cheese used in salads, breads, and entrées. In Greece, this cheese is usually made from ewe's or goat's milk; in the United States it is made from cow's milk.

Fontina. This cheese, which comes from Italy, is made either from cow's or ewe's milk. In the United States it is always made from cow's milk.

Gavot. This cheese is prepared from ewe's, cow's, or goat's milk.

Kassari. A snappy flavored cheese with a golden appearance, it is a good substitute for Parmesan cheese in recipes. This cheese, imported from Greece, is manufactured from ewe's or goat's milk.

Kefalotysi. Another cheese from Greece, Kefalotysi is a hard cheese used mostly for grating. This cheese is produced from either ewe's or goat's milk. Surprisingly, this cheese is also produced in the Ozark region of Arkansas.

Pecorino. Also known as Pecorino Romano, Pecorino Dolco, Pecorino Grosetto, this cheese comes from Italy. All varieties are made only from ewe's milk.

Romano. See Pecorino.

Roquefort. This cheese, which has a very pronounced taste, is used in salads, dressings, and cheese spreads. Imported from France, it is produced from raw ewe's milk.

Sardo Romano. Made from a mixture of cow's and ewe's milk, this cheese is not satisfactory for use in the recipes of this book.

Serra de Estralla. This cheese is manufactured exclusively from ewe's milk. Sometimes it may contain goat's milk.

Tignaid. A cheese made entirely from ewe's or goat's milk.

Touloumiso. This cheese is imported from Greece. The ingredients found in this cheese are identical to those found in Feta cheese.

Valdeblore. Produced in France, this mild cheese is used as an appetizer or as a condiment for many dishes.

Cheeses made from goat's milk

Bucheron. A French imported cheese with a very goaty taste.

Capricette. Another French import, this cheese is smooth with a tangy taste.

Chevrotins. Also known as Chevret cheeses, these goat cheeses are popular gourmet items and thus expensive. The Chevrotins that are pure goat's milk are: Chevret de Comme, Chevret de Moulins, Chevret de Souvigny.

Feta. A cheese from Greece, which is made from ewe's milk and sometimes goat's milk.

Jonchee Niortaise. This is a fresh goat's milk cheese. It is used in sweet desserts such as cheesecakes.

La Banion. A French import, this cheese has a slightly nutty flavor.

La Mothe-Saint-Héray. A cheese that an individual just starting to taste goat cheeses should not start with. This cheese has a definite bite to it.

Montrachet. This French imported cheese is mild and creamy. It is usually served at the end of a meal with fruit.

Persillés Des Aravio. This is a very tangy and sharp cheese. It is good as an appetizer.

Poivre-d'Ane. Another French import, this cheese is mild and is seasoned with herbs. Beware—this cheese is sometimes mixed with cow's milk.

Roila. A cheese made exclusively from goat's or ewe's milk.

Teleme. Also known as Brandza de Braila, this cheese is produced from fresh goat's or ewe's milk.

Valencay. Made from raw goat's milk, this cheese has a slightly nutty taste.

EGGS

The importance of eggs as a complete protein is marred by the fact that they contain as much fat as they do protein (most of the fat is in the yolk). Eggs are also known for their allergy potential. Generally, this is due to the protein found in the egg white. Until eggs are ruled out as allergy-causing, the cook should use the egg substitutes listed in Appendix A. (NOTE: Some of the commerical brands listed contain milk by-products.)

FISH

Fish, especially white fish (turbot, snapper, sole, cod, trout), is another complete protein food. Unlike meat, it contains very little fat. Fatty fish (salmon, herring, mackeral, tuna) contain a little more fat than white fish, but are still an immense improvement over red meat. Shellfish (oysters, crab, lobster, scallops, shrimp), known for their allergenic properties, will not be found in any recipes in this book.

FLOURS

Arrowroot. A flour used as a thickening agent that is usually found in the spice section of most supermarkets.

Potato Flour. A heavy flour with a distinctive taste of its own. Most health food stores carry it. If necessary, (pure) mashed potatoes could be substituted. Potato flour is a good source of phosphorous, calcium, sodium, and iron. It is an excellent source of potassium.

Potato Starch. A very light flour that is an excellent ingredient for sponge cake, muffins, and pancakes. Most supermarkets carry it.

Rice Flour. A very grainy dry flour. Adding a moisture retaining flour such as potato flour or soy flour helps with the texture of items baked with rice flour. It can be found in most health food stores.

Rice Baking Mix. A gluten-free mix to be used like Bisquick. It can be found in most health food stores.

Soy Flour. Soy flour is a highly concentrated vegetable protein derived from soybeans. It has a yellowish color and nutty taste. It is a rich source of protein, Vitamin B, calcium, potassium, and iron. It will add moisture to dry flours in baking and is an excellent addition to cakes, pie crusts, breads, and rolls.

Tapioca. Tapioca flour is a good source of phosphorous, potassium, calcium, and magnesium. The easiest form of tapioca to find is quick tapioca. Tapioca starch is a little harder to find. Use it to replace cornstarch for thickening. Do not overheat tapioca for it will lose its thickening ability.

GRAINS

Buckwheat (Kasha). Buckwheat is a grain cultivated for flour or groats. It can be eaten as a cereal or cooked like rice. It is a good source of phosphorous and potassium. Most health food stores carry it.

Millet. This grain is produced in the United States and Europe for its small edible seeds. Its protein content is higher than barley or corn. It is a good fiber source, and is extremely rich in phosphorous, potassium, and magnesium.

Rice. Types of rice:

Brown rice. This is a vitamin rich food because the bran layer has not been removed. Brown rice contains a rich supply of Vitamin B, calcium, phosphorous, and iron.

White rice. This rice loses more than 2 percent of its protein and all of its thiamine because the hull and the bran are removed by polishing. However, enriched rice has a premix of vitamins (especially thiamine) and iron added to it. Converted rice undergoes a similar manufacturing process, but is left with a higher vitamin content than white rice.

Risotto. This is a short-grain rice of Italian origin. It will not become soggy with slow cooking. Most Italian markets carry it.

HERBS AND SPICES

Any herb or spice might be a potential cause of an allergy. This book does use *some* herbs and spices. It is suggested that when such herbs are used that they are fresh or freshly dried.

Basil. This herb is a member of the mint family. It has a pleasant sweet flavor. Its uses are many, especially in stews, beans, and vegetables. Soups, salads, poultry, and meats are more appealing with this seasoning.

Bay Leaves. This mild herb from the European Bay or Laurel and from the California Bay is frequently used to season all types of meats, vegetables, soups, relishes, poultry, and stuffings.

Capers. This seasoning is a bud off a Mediterranean plant belonging to the mustard family. Capers are often found in Italian dishes. They are either pickled or preserved in salt.

Fennel Seed. This is a spice with a distinctive flavor, not unlike licorice. It originated from India and parts of Bulgaria. The seeds are used in salads, vegetable dishes, and fish dishes, and to spice up rolls and breads.

Dill. This seasoning in seed or dried weed form has a delightful flavor that tastes somewhat like parsley yet with a little more tang. Dill goes with fish, poultry, salads, and sauces. Traditionally, it is used between layers of cucumber in brine to make dill pickles.

Italian Seasoning. A mixture of dried herbs containing oregano, marjoram, thyme, savory, basil, rosemary, and sage. It is usually found in the spice section of most markets.

Marjoram. Sweet marjoram is a subtle herb with a pleasing taste that enhances a food without altering the food's flavor. This herb is used for sauces, soups, salads, meats, stuffings and fish.

Mint. An herb with the flavor of spearmint, mint does wonders for lamb dishes. It will also enhance the flavor of vegetables, salads, meat broths, teas, and ices.

Oregano. An herb known as "joy of the mountain," oregano is indispensible in Italian, Spanish, and Greek dishes. It can be used in meat dishes, beans, soups, and sauces.

Parsley. This herb with its crisp leaves is used extensively as a garnish and seasoning. It has the added benefit of being a rich source of Vitamins C and A, and of iron.

Rosemary. Rosemary is an evergreen often found growing along the coast of the Mediterranean. It is an herb with a powerful flavor that enriches meat dishes, sauces, greens, and stuffings.

Sage. Sage is a culinary herb that is satisfactory for stuffings, stews, and bean dishes. It should never be used alone, but with thyme or basil.

Tarragon. Tarragon is an invaluable herb for a fish sauce, for it removes the fishy odor and leaves a fresh, pleasant flavor. It is also used for poultry sauces, stews, meats, soups, and dressings. Tarragon is the most important seasoning for tartar sauce.

Thyme. Thyme is an evergreen with a strong, sweet flavor. It is a most versatile herb and can be found in soups, sauces, stuffings, spreads, meats, fish, poultry, and dressings. It is usually used in tomato dishes or dishes with tomato sauce.

LIQUIDS

Soy Milk. Soy milk has been recommended by physicians for years to patients who are allergic to cow's milk. Soy milk is low in fat and carbohydrates. It is rich in thiamine and niacine.

Non-citrus Juices. Examples of such juices are "pure" apple juice, pear, apricot, and cranberry juice.

MEATS

Lamb and Beef. Both lamb and beef contain protein, B vitamins, and iron. Like dairy products, meats are complete protein foods. Unfortunately, they are also high in saturated fats. When selecting a meat (lamb or beef) choose a lean meat. When selecting a cured meat choose a Kosher brand. Kosher meats do not have any milk or milk by-products in the meat. When preparing the meat, be sure that all meats are cooked to at least a pink color. Rare meats tend to cause headaches.

NUTS

Almonds. Although the almond really belongs to the plum family, it is still classified as a nut. Almonds are rich in protein and unsaturated fats. Almonds contain high amounts of phosphorus, potassium, and calcium. When almonds are referred to in the recipe section, the almonds should be roasted or toasted to remove any oil or extracts known for their allergenic properties.

Pine Nuts. Pine nuts are another mislabeled nut. Pine nuts are really seeds of the Stone Pine tree. Rich in iron, potassium, and phosphorous, these "nuts" are 31 percent protein. Pine nuts are used in Italian, Greek and Middle Eastern cooking. These seeds are about ½ inch long with a delicate flavor that enhances most entrées.

OILS AND MARGARINES

Olive Oil. This monounsaturated oil contains only 10 percent of the necessary fatty acid, linoleic acid. It also has more calories than butter or lard. This oil will be found in Italian, Greek, and other Mediterranean dishes. Use it sparingly.

Safflower Oil (or margarine). This is a cold, pressed, polyunsaturated natural oil, containing 70–80 percent of the necessary fatty acid, linoleic acid. Safflower oil is a good source of Vitamin E.

Soybean Oil (or margarine). This is another polyunsaturated oil with 60 percent linoleic acid. Soybean oil is a good source of lecithin and Vitamin E.

Sesame Oil. This polyunsaturated oil is used only sparingly with other oils. It is found mostly in Oriental and Indonesian dishes.

Sesame Seed Oil. This is a cold, pressed, polyunsaturated natural oil found in most health food stores.

POULTRY

Turkey and Chicken. Another complete protein food, fowl is low in saturated fats. This book requests that male birds be used in most recipe dishes.

SOYBEAN PRODUCTS AND SEASONINGS

Miso. Known also as bean curd paste, miso is a high-protein seasoning produced from soybeans. Like yoghurt, it contains lactobacillus and other healthful bacteria regarded as beneficial to the intestine. The Japanese use it as a basic staple as it is a concentrated source of protein. Miso is used along with tamari-like bouillon in soups and stews, and like Worcestershire in sauces, dressings, and dips. Brown rice miso is the miso of choice. It has a deep, rich flavor and a pleasant fragrance. This particular type of miso contains 12–14 percent protein and is relatively easy to find.

Tamari. Tamari is a seasoning that is much richer than most soy sauces. Use it sparingly. The variety used in this book does not contain wheat. Be sure to check the labels.

Tofu. Also known as soybean curd, this is made from the only legume that is a complete protein. It is a common food of the traditional Oriental diet and often referred to as "the meat without a bone."

SWEETENERS

Carob. Carob, fruit of an evergreen tree known as St. Jolen, is a natural sweetener. It is rich in Vitamin A and B, and minerals. It can be used as a replacement for cocoa and chocolate.

Honey. Honey is almost twice as sweet as cane or beet sugar. Smaller amounts are needed for sweetening. However, the sources of honey are so variable as to severely limit its uses in hypoallergenic cooking.

Molasses (blackstrap). This is the last substance left after the extraction of sugar from the sugar cane. It is a rich source of vitamins and minerals, especially iron.

Maple Syrup. This is usually a solution of dissolved sugar with maple extract. Maple syrup in its pure form can be found but it is expensive.

Sugar. Sugar is a sweet, crystalline substance obtained from the juice of the sugar cane or sugar beet. It is a major carbohydrate source lacking any protein, vitamins, or minerals.

RECOMMENDED RECIPES FOR TESTING

Milk

Baked Lamb Chops, 74–75
Carob Mousse II, 180
Cream Cheese Frosting, 183
Eggplant and Onion Soup, 41–42
Lima Bean Casserole, 100
Nachos, 35
Potato and Onion Soup, 43
Skillet Zucchini, 133
Turkey Goulash, 95
Vegetarian Pizza, 104

Eggs

Buckwheat Loaf, 65
Carrot Lamb Loaf, 76
Carrot Nut Cake, 171
Maple Syrup Cake, 173
Nature's Macaroons, 190
Romano Sole, 55
Roquefort Cheese Mold, 111
Spinach Pie, 101
Squash Pie, 102
Tuna Patties, 61
Zucchini Salad, 146

RECOMMENDED ALLERGY COOKBOOKS

Carter, Patricia. *Allergy Cookbook*. Horn Church, England: Ian Henry Publications, England State Mutual Bank, 1981.

Emerling, Carol, and Eugene O. Jonchers. *The Allergy Cookbook*. Garden City, New York: Doubleday & Co., 1969.

Frazier, Claude, *Coping with Food Allergy*. New York: Quadrangle, 1974.

Lacey, Suzanne S. *The Allergic Person's Cookbook*. Springfield, Illinois: Charles C. Thomas, 1981.

Majors, Judith S. *Sugar Free That's Me*. New York: Ballantine Books, 1980.

Mandell, Marshall, and Gare, Fran. *Dr. Mandell's Allergy Free Cookbook*. New York: Pocket Books, 1981.

Rudoff, Carol. *The Allergy Baker: A Collection of Wheat-Free, Milk-Free, Egg-Free, Corn-Free, and Soy-Free Recipes*. Menlo Park, California: Prologue Publications, 1980.

Shattuck, Ruth R. *Creative Cooking Without Wheat, Milk, and Eggs*. South Brunswick, New York: A. S. Barnes, 1973.

Thomas, Linda. *Caring and Cooking for the Allergic Child*. New York: Sterling Publishing Co., 1980.

BIBLIOGRAPHY

BOOKS

Androque, Pierre. *The Complete Encyclopedia of French Cheese.* New York: Harper's Magazine Press, 1973.

Bottomley, H. W. *Allergy: Its Treatment and Care.* New York: Funk and Wagnalls, 1969.

Brainard, John B. *Control of Migraine.* New York: W. W. Norton & Company, Inc., 1977.

Emerling, Carol, and Eugene O. Jonchers. *The Allergy Cookbook.* Garden City, New York: Doubleday & Co., 1969.

Forster, Gertrude B. *Herbs for Every Garden.* New York: E. P. Dutton & Co., Inc., 1966.

Frazier, Claude A. *Coping with Food Allergy.* New York: Quadrangle, 1974.

———. *Parents Guide to Allergy in Children.* New York: Grossett and Dunlap, 1978.

Giannini, Allen V. *The Best Guide to Allergy.* New York: Appleton-Century-Crofts, 1981.

Hamrick, Becky, and S. L. Wiesenfeld, M.D. *The Egg-Free, Milk-Free, Wheat-Free Cookbook.* New York: Harper & Row, 1981.

Hewitt, Jean. *Natural Foods Cookbook.* New York: Avon, 1971.

Hills, Hilda Chevy. *Good Food, Gluten-Free.* New Canaan, Connecticut: Keats Publishings, Inc., 1976.

Jones, Dorothea Van Gundy. *Soybean Cookbook.* New York: Arc Books, 1968.

Kadans, Joseph M. *The Encyclopedia of Fruits, Vegetables, Nuts, and Seeds for Healthful Living.* West Nyak, New York: Parker Publishing Company, Inc., 1974.

Kirchmann, John D. ed. *Nutrition Almanac.* New York: McGraw-Hill Book Company, 1979.

Pearl, Anita. *Completely Cheese, The Cheeselover's Companion.* New York: Jonathan David Publishers, Inc., 1978.

Rapport, Howard G., and Shirley Motter Linde. *The Complete Allergy Guide.* New York: Simon & Schuster, 1970.

Sainsburg, Isobel S. *The Milk-Free and Milk/Egg-Free Cookbook.* New York: Arco Publishing, 1979.

Seddon, George, and Jackie Burrow. *The Natural Food Book.* New York: Rand McNally, 1977.

The Settlement Cookbook. New York: Simon & Schuster, 1954.

Shattuch, Ruth R. *Creative Cooking Without Wheat, Milk and Eggs.* South Brunswick, New York: A.S. Barnes & Company, 1976.

Shurtleff, William, and Akiko Aoyagi. *The Book of Miso.* Brookline, Massachusetts: Autumn Press, 1976.

Speer, Frederick. *Food Allergy.* Littleton, Massachusetts: PSG Publishing Company, Inc., 1979.

Taube, Louis E. *Food Allergy and the Allergy Patient.* Springfield, Illinois: Charles C. Thomas Publisher, 1978.

Zierbel, Runa, and Victor Zierbel. *The Vegetarian Family.* Englewood Cliffs, New Jersey: Prentice-Hall, Inc., 1978.

ARTICLES

"Immunological Assays for Coeliac Disease." *Lancet,* (May 23, 1981): 1156–9.

Lebenthal, Emanual, M.D., and David Branski, M.D. "Childhood Celiac Disease —a Reappraisal." *Journal of Pediatrics,* 98: 5 (May 1981): 681–690.

Neild, G. H. "Food Allergies." *Lancet,* (April 11, 1981): 811–812.

INDEX

Risotto, 1, 116, 212
Roquefort cheese, 210
  biscuits, 166–167
  dressing
    Italian style, 149
    I, 148
    II, 148
  mold, 111–112
  salad, and tomato, 143–144
Runny nose, 3
Runting, 5
Rye, 10

S

Safflower
  margarine, 9, 215
  oil, 2, 215
Salad(s)
  apple nut slaw, 144
  artichoke-spinach, 135
  avocado, 136
    provençal, 137
  banana
    -apple, 137
    fruit mold, 137–138
  bean supreme, 138
  beet, 135
  carrot-raisin, 136
  chicken, Chinese, 138–139
  cranberry apple, 139
  cucumber platter, 139
  Feta, 140
  fruit, 140
    nutty, 136
  garbanzo-kidney bean, 141
  Greek, 141
  green, 142
  mushroom-cucumber, 142
  pachadi, 143
  potato, 143
  Roquefort and tomato, 143–144
  spinach-sesame, Oriental, 142
  tabbouléh, 144
  turkey, 145
  Waldorf, 145
  zucchini, 146
Salad dressing
  dillweed, 149
  French
    I, 147
    II, 147

Greek, 150
  Italian, curried, 151
  mayonnaise
    I, eggless, 149
    II, eggless, 150
  miso, 154
  mustard, 152
  Roquefort
    Italian-style, 149
    I, 148
    II, 148
  tahini sauce, 151
  tarragon, 150
  vinaigrette, 148
Salmon (see Fish), 8
Salt, 4
  headache-free, seasoned, 154
Sauce
  béchamel, 153
  cheese, 109
  dessert (see Dessert sauce)
  miso, prepared, 154
  mushroom, 153
  tahini, 151
  tartar, 152
  white
    I, 151
    II, 152
Sauerkraut, 4
Scotch, 4
Seasonings (see also Herbs and
    Spices), 9
  bouquet garni, 154
  coconut stock, 154
  mint, dried, 153
  salt, headache-free, 154
Sesame seed(s), 9, 215
  candy
    almond I, 190–191
    almond II, 191
  cookies, 190
  meatloaf, 66
  oil, 9, 215
Sfeeha, meat pie, 81–82
Shellfish (see Crustaceans)
Shortening, 11
Sinus, 4
Sole (see Fish)
Snapper (see Fish)
Soup(s)
  beef stock, 37
  borsch, Russian, 38

Z

Zucchini
  boats, 106–107
  fritters, 113
  grilled, cheesy, 133
  salad, 146
  skillet, 133
  soup, 48–49